COVID-19 in the Commonwealth

2020 was the first year of the COVID-19 pandemic, the most significant global pandemic since the 'Spanish flu' in 1918–1919. This book provides an analysis of the experience of the COVID-19 pandemic in a range of Commonwealth countries during 2020, covering public health, political, economic and international aspects.

The Commonwealth, within which about one quarter of the world's population resides, provides a cross-section of the global experience of COVID-19. The Commonwealth ranges from highly populated countries such as India and Nigeria, to small island states and territories, encompassing also advanced industrialised countries and developing countries. The grouping also extends into many different regions of the world: Africa, South and Southeast Asia, Europe, the Americas and Oceania. In the first year of the pandemic, vaccines were still under development and national response strategies chosen by Commonwealth countries were diverse, spanning eradication, elimination, suppression and mitigation. The chapters in this book show the ways in which governments from a selection of Commonwealth countries responded to the multiple dimensions of the crisis, pointing to the factors that led to effective or less effective policies.

This book originally appeared as a special issue of *The Round Table: The Commonwealth Journal of International Affairs*.

Derek McDougall specialises in Asia-Pacific international politics, with particular reference to Australian engagement. He is the author of *Asia-Pacific in World Politics* (2016). He is a frequent contributor to *The Round Table: The Commonwealth Journal of International Affairs* and serves on the journal's international advisory board.

Suan Ee Ong has an academic background in political science and public health. She is a senior researcher and member of senior management at Research for Impact, a Singapore-based social, behavioural and health research organisation. She also holds honorary fellowships at the National University of Singapore's School of Public Health and the Galen Centre for Health and Social Policy in Malaysia.

COVID-19 in the Commonwealth

Edited by
Derek McDougall and Suan Ee Ong

Routledge
Taylor & Francis Group
LONDON AND NEW YORK

First published 2023
by Routledge
4 Park Square, Milton Park, Abingdon, Oxon OX14 4RN

and by Routledge
605 Third Avenue, New York, NY 10158

Routledge is an imprint of the Taylor & Francis Group, an informa business

British Library Cataloguing in Publication Data
A catalogue record for this book is available from the British Library

ISBN13: 978-1-032-37666-0 (hbk)
ISBN13: 978-1-032-37667-7 (pbk)
ISBN13: 978-1-003-34129-1 (ebk)

DOI: 10.4324/9781003341291

Typeset in Minion Pro
by Newgen Publishing UK

Publisher's Note
The publisher accepts responsibility for any inconsistencies that may have arisen during the conversion of this book from journal articles to book chapters, namely the inclusion of journal terminology.

Contents

Citation Information

The following chapters were originally published in *The Round Table: The Commonwealth Journal of International Affairs*, volume 110, issue 1 (2021). When citing this material, please use the original page numbering for each article, as follows:

Chapter 1
In, but not of, Africa: a divided South Africa faces COVID-19
Steven Friedman
The Round Table: The Commonwealth Journal of International Affairs, volume 110, issue 1 (2021), pp. 16–30

Chapter 2
Canada and COVID-19: the longer-term geopolitical implications
Kim Richard Nossal
The Round Table: The Commonwealth Journal of International Affairs, volume 110, issue 1 (2021), pp. 31–45

Chapter 3
India's domestic and foreign policy responses to COVID-19
Pradeep Taneja and Azad Singh Bali
The Round Table: The Commonwealth Journal of International Affairs, volume 110, issue 1 (2021), pp. 46–61

Chapter 4
COVID-19, Brexit and the United Kingdom – a year of uncertainty
Julie Smith
The Round Table: The Commonwealth Journal of International Affairs, volume 110, issue 1 (2021), pp. 62–75

Chapter 5
COVID-19 in Nigeria
Noo Saro-Wiwa
The Round Table: The Commonwealth Journal of International Affairs, volume 110, issue 1 (2021), pp. 76–83

Chapter 6

Malaysia, Myanmar and Singapore: common threads, divergences, and lessons learned in responding to the COVID-19 pandemic
Kyaw San Wai, Wai Yee Krystal Khine, Jane Mingjie Lim, Pearlyn Hui Min Neo, Rayner Kay Jin Tan and Suan Ee Ong
The Round Table: The Commonwealth Journal of International Affairs, volume 110, issue 1 (2021), pp. 84–98

Chapter 7

Impacts of COVID-19 in the Commonwealth Caribbean: key lessons
Jessica Byron, Jacqueline Laguardia Martinez, Annita Montoute and Keron Niles
The Round Table: The Commonwealth Journal of International Affairs, volume 110, issue 1 (2021), pp. 99–119

Chapter 8

Australia and New Zealand: the pandemic Down Under
Derek McDougall
The Round Table: The Commonwealth Journal of International Affairs, volume 110, issue 1 (2021), pp. 120–137

Chapter 9

COVID-19 in the Pacific Island Commonwealth: microstates managing a macro-challenge
Richard Herr
The Round Table: The Commonwealth Journal of International Affairs, volume 110, issue 1 (2021), pp. 138–148

Chapter 10

COVID-19 and tourism in Pacific SIDS: lessons from Fiji, Vanuatu and Samoa?
John Connell
The Round Table: The Commonwealth Journal of International Affairs, volume 110, issue 1 (2021), pp. 149–158

Chapter 11

COVID-19 and the British Overseas Territories: a comparative view
Matthew C. Benwell, Peter Clegg and Alasdair Pinkerton
The Round Table: The Commonwealth Journal of International Affairs, volume 110, issue 1 (2021), pp. 159–170

Notes on Contributors

Azad Singh Bali, School of Politics and International Relations and the Crawford School of Public Policy, Australian National University, Canberra, Australia.

Matthew C. Benwell, School of Geography, Politics and Sociology, Newcastle University, Newcastle upon Tyne, UK.

Jessica Byron, Institute of International Relations, The University of the West Indies, St. Augustine, West Indies.

Peter Clegg, Department of Health and Social Sciences, University of the West of England, Bristol, UK.

John Connell, School of Geosciences, University of Sydney, Sydney, Australia.

Steven Friedman, Faculty of Humanities, University of Johannesburg, Johannesburg, South Africa.

Richard Herr, Faculty of Law, University of Tasmania, Hobart, Tasmania, Australia.

Wai Yee Krystal Khine, Lee Kuan Yew School of Public Policy, National University of Singapore, Singapore.

Jane Mingjie Lim, Saw Swee Hock School of Public Health, National University of Singapore and National University Health System, Singapore.

Jacqueline Laguardia Martinez, Institute of International Relations, The University of the West Indies, St. Augustine, West Indies.

Derek McDougall, School of Social and Political Sciences, University of Melbourne, Melbourne, Australia.

Annita Montoute, Institute of International Relations, The University of the West Indies, St. Augustine, West Indies.

Pearlyn Hui Min Neo, Saw Swee Hock School of Public Health, National University of Singapore, Singapore.

Keron Niles, Institute of International Relations, The University of the West Indies, St. Augustine, West Indies.

Kim Richard Nossal, Department of Political Studies, Queen's University, Kingston, Ontario, Canada.

Suan Ee Ong, Research for Impact, Singapore; Saw Swee Hock School of Public Health, National University of Singapore, Singapore; Galen Centre for Health and Social Policy, Kuala Lumpur, Malaysia.

Alasdair Pinkerton, Department of Geography, Royal Holloway, University of London, Surrey, UK.

Noo Saro-Wiwa, Independent Writer and Journaist, Port Harcourt, Nigeria.

Julie Smith, Department of Politics and International Studies, University of Cambridge, Cambridge, UK; Fellow in Politics, Robinson College, University of Cambridge, Cambridge, UK.

Rayner Kay Jin Tan, Saw Swee Hock School of Public Health, National University of Singapore and National University Health, System, Singapore; University of North Carolina Project-China, China.

Pradeep Taneja, School of Social and Political Sciences, University of Melbourne, Melbourne, Australia.

Kyaw San Wai, Myanmar Health and Development Consortium, Yangon, Myanmar; MSc (Distance) Student, London School of Hygiene and Tropical Medicine, University of London, London, UK.

Introduction: COVID-19 in the Commonwealth

Derek McDougall and Suan Ee Ong

[The Introduction as it originally appeared in *The Round Table*, vol. 110, no. 1 (2021) reflected the experience of COVID-19 in the Commonwealth during 2020. The text has been slightly modified to allow for the book version being published approximately two years later. Please note that all chapters remain the same as they were as articles in the special issue, providing assessments relating to the different countries, territories and regions as of the end of 2020.]

The year 2020 was the year of the COVID-19 pandemic, an *annus horribilis.* After the first reported outbreak of the novel coronavirus in Wuhan, China in December 2019, the virus spread around the world, affecting virtually all countries but with varying impacts. By year's end, the number of cases recorded globally was about 75 million, with deaths totalling about 1.7 million. The top five affected countries by total case numbers were the United States, India, Brazil, Russia and France (Worldometer, 17 December 2020). In relative terms (using number of cases per million people), the worst affected countries with populations over 10 million were the Czech Republic, Belgium and the United States, in descending order. The United States, with a population of about 333 million, recorded 17.4 million cases and 314,577 deaths as of 17 December 2020.[1] The way the pandemic evolved raises questions about why and how countries responded and how effective their policies were.

Given this book is entitled *COVID-19 in the Commonwealth*, we need to ask what the value of a Commonwealth perspective is on these general issues concerning the pandemic. As with many other global issues, the value of a Commonwealth perspective is that it provides a cross-section of the pandemic experience across the whole world, covering developed and developing countries (and different types within those broad categories), established and emerging powers, some of the most populous countries in different regions, as well as small states and territories. The focus of this book is on countries that are members of the Commonwealth (including dependent territories), rather than on the role of the Commonwealth of Nations or the Commonwealth Secretariat more specifically.

The chapters in this book cover several significant countries and regions within the Commonwealth, without purporting to be comprehensive. There is a strong emphasis on small island states and territories (four chapters), but the Commonwealth itself also has that emphasis (32 of 56 members are defined as small states, of which 24 are small island states, or 27 if Belize, Guyana and Brunei Darussalam are included). The authors come from different parts of the Commonwealth, but Australia is undoubtedly overrepresented, suggesting a bias towards an Antipodean view of the Commonwealth. Australia clearly has a strong focus on the Pacific island countries and Southeast Asia, while also having important links to the United Kingdom and Canada as old Commonwealth countries, and to India as both an emerging power and a prominent Commonwealth member.

The relative impact of COVID-19 varied greatly across the Commonwealth states and dependent territories – from Gibraltar (ranked 32nd by Worldometer, total cases in relation to population, 17 December 2020) to Vanuatu (ranked 215th, bottom of the list of countries and territories). Among the countries covered in this book (other than regions and the British overseas territories) the ranking was the United Kingdom (46th), South Africa (77th), Canada (87th), Singapore (96th), India (107th), Malaysia (127th), Myanmar (not a Commonwealth member) (135th), Australia (152nd) and New Zealand (180th). Taking Papua New Guinea and Jamaica as the largest of the Commonwealth Pacific island countries (PICs) and the Commonwealth Caribbean respectively, the ranking is 201st (PNG) and 122nd (Jamaica).

General issues

On the assumption that the Commonwealth countries and territories provide a cross section of the world, it is helpful to read the various articles from the perspective of how they assess responses to the key issues arising from the pandemic. The emphasis across chapters will vary, with some chapters attempting to be comprehensive, while other articles focus more on particular aspects. The key issues covered are public health responses, economic responses and consequences, the relevance of domestic politics, and the pandemic's impact on geopolitics.

Public health responses

From a public health perspective, COVID-19 stretched national health systems to their limits. All countries and territories featured in this book grappled with the same slate of fundamental public health challenges: testing, tracing, and isolation of potentially exposed or infected individuals, suppressing transmission in the general population, protecting healthcare workers, preventing patients' progression to severe disease or death, keeping up with the latest developments in drug, treatment and vaccine technologies, and maintaining delivery of essential health and social care services. Despite these shared challenges, initial public health responses to the pandemic reflected differences at the confluence of political will, sociocultural acceptability, disease burden, health system resilience, and ability to amass, deploy and distribute financial and human resources.

For a pandemic occurring in the modern era of globalisation, information exchange, and movement of persons and goods, a main challenge for national governments was what strategy to choose to manage COVID-19. In the early days of the pandemic, some countries elected to use mitigation strategies to manage the pandemic's negative health impacts, in some instances (Sweden, with some initial discussion also in the United Kingdom) with the aim of achieving herd immunity (i.e., a form of indirect protection from an infectious disease that happens when a sufficient proportion of the population (about 70 per cent) has become immune to the infection through previous infections or vaccination). However, it was not long until COVID-19 cases began overwhelming health systems, prompting a shift towards a situation where a range of suppression strategies emerged, focused on drastically reducing transmission to the point that sustained, community transmission was no longer possible. To do this, some countries relied more heavily on traditional containment measures (i.e., quarantines, lockdowns) than did others; suppression varied between 'hard' and 'soft' versions.

In relation to strategies, a key question that repeatedly came to the fore was 'what determines the effectiveness of a public health response to COVID-19?' The answer, for better or for worse, was, 'it depends'. The inherent political and resource differences across the countries featured in this book and how these characteristics interacted with public health responses and populations' sociocultural leanings were evidence that there is no one-size-fits-all, replicable, effective method to manage COVID-19. Two notable examples of this were: (i) Singapore and the way in which its ability to implement rapidly border closures, temperature screenings and other public health measures was facilitated by its small size, pragmatic government and largely law-abiding population; and (ii) New Zealand's ambitious 'hard' suppression strategy, close to elimination, grounded in decisive leadership, early action, highly functioning public health infrastructure, 'remote' island location, low population density and a cooperative public.

The public health landscape substantially shifted at the end of 2020 with the announcement of efficacious vaccines developed by pharmaceutical companies Pfizer and Moderna, with other players like Johnson and Johnson, Sinovac and AstraZeneca not far behind. From this time the global COVID-19 discourse was dominated by vaccination concerns that were common to all countries affected by the pandemic, including safety, side effects, vaccine hesitancy, production, access, supply chain management, distribution and prioritisation. In December 2020 the United Kingdom began rolling out its nationwide vaccination programme, targeting the immunisation of 25 million people in selected groups including the elderly, frontline health and social care workers, and the clinically vulnerable (Triggle, 2020). The other Commonwealth countries featured in this book, from Canada to Malaysia, were also in the midst of developing and executing their national COVID-19 vaccination plans. Although vaccine news gave rise to a wave of optimism and growing research projecting the optimal proportions of the population who needed to be vaccinated in order to achieve herd immunity, evidence around immunity to COVID-19, including duration, strength, and differentiation by subpopulations by clinical risk profiles, was still emerging at the end of 2020.

Economic responses and consequences

Given that COVID-19 necessitated curtailing proximity of people-to-people interactions, with restrictions varying depending on the severity of the pandemic in each setting and different national governments' policy positions, clearly, there was a huge economic impact. Economic activity of various kinds was severely reduced. With many occupations, people were required to work from home. Major economic sectors, most notably hospitality and tourism, either shut down completely or closed temporarily; these sectors continued to struggle as governments lifted and re-imposed lockdowns in various forms in response to changing infection numbers. With international and domestic travel restricted, aviation sectors in many countries required government support to survive. Immigration programmes largely ceased, and international student flows became much more difficult. Schools and universities were closed in many countries for long periods, with many making major operational shifts towards comprehensive virtual learning.

Given the onset of recession as a result of the pandemic, most governments pursued Keynesian policies in response, regarding themselves as playing the leading role in ensuring economic survival and long-term recovery. This involved assuming high levels of debt, making the response in many circumstances comparable to the kind of debt governments took on during the world wars. Businesses received direct support, and there were major programmes to assist the unemployed. As such, economically stronger developed countries were in a better position to undertake these interventionist policies than were developing countries, particularly the poorer ones.

Countries that responded strongly to COVID-19 through their public health policies, enabling a return to 'normal' life sooner rather than later, were in a better position to pursue economic recovery than those responding slowly and less effectively. Going beyond immediate recovery, issues were posed about how COVID-19 would affect economies in the long term, with the high levels of debt needing to be serviced. Were policies of austerity likely, or would the economic stimulus provided by the Keynesian policies be sufficient to enable a return to an era of growth?

The relevance of domestic politics

Decisions in response to the health and economic aspects of the pandemic were made by national and local governments. Different political arrangements had an influence on the way in which pandemic issues were handled. Some political environments were more complex than others. Federal systems (e.g., Canada and Australia) involve overlapping jurisdictions; complexity can also exist with devolved administrations (e.g., the United Kingdom). Unitary systems can appear more straightforward. However, it is possible to achieve a high level of cooperation in a federation. Likewise, there can be significant conflict within a unitary system.

As the pandemic progressed, there were tensions in some countries along a left–right spectrum. Left-leaning governments and parties were more likely to favour more restrictive health measures and strong economic stimulus programmes. Meanwhile, on the right, there was more pressure to move quickly to ease lockdowns and a greater sensitivity to business concerns. This is not to say that there was not a lot of overlap; the differences were ones of emphasis.

COVID-19 was a test of the capacity of different systems to cope with a major crisis. This was not just a matter of the political arrangements as such but also involved the bureaucratic and technical resources required to respond effectively to a pandemic.

The impact on geopolitics

Responding to COVID-19 involved not just decisions by individual governments. By definition, a pandemic is international in scope. While the spread of the pandemic had an international context, there was also an international response. The World Health Organization (WHO), despite some criticism of its supposedly slow reactions in the initial phase of the pandemic, played a key role throughout in monitoring the pandemic and advising governments, without necessarily playing a leading role. Much commentary has suggested that the pandemic led to an increased emphasis on states prioritising their own interests, 'vaccine nationalism' being a good example with governments mainly concerned about the protection of their own citizens and residents – although not necessarily exclusively so.

In terms of geopolitics, one of the impacts of COVID-19 was that states that fared better in combating the virus might enhance their geopolitical position. Such an outcome depended on how any given state compared with its neighbours and the other countries with which it had significant interactions. In the COVID-19 environment, there might be situations arising that gave some states additional leverage. Among the countries covered in this book, Australia and New Zealand might have enhanced their positions vis-à-vis their South Pacific neighbours. Canada, despite managing COVID-19 better than the United States, might have experienced some geopolitical decline, largely because of its proximity to the United States (affected not just by the poor performance of the United States in relation to COVID, but by the undermining of multilateralism under the Trump administration). Conversely, COVID-19 appeared to improve India's position within South Asia in 2020, with India playing the key role in that region's response to the pandemic (through the South Asian Association of Regional Cooperation [SAARC]), as well as leading globally through the Non-aligned Movement and the G-20.

Small island states and territories

As indicated, this book has some focus on small island states and territories, with one chapter on the Commonwealth Caribbean, two on the PICs, and one on the UK overseas territories. The general issues that have been raised can also be addressed in this context, but is there anything that can be said pertaining specifically to these polities? During 2020 a picture emerged of both vulnerability and resilience.

Although Gibraltar (not an island) was actually the worst affected of any Commonwealth country or Commonwealth-linked territory (total cases per capita, as previously indicated), overall, the small island states and territories did relatively well in controlling the spread of COVID-19. In the case of the PICs and many of the UK overseas territories, this capacity for control was facilitated by their isolated geographical location. The most severe impacts of the pandemic on these island states and territories were economic, as many of these polities were highly dependent on tourism and remittances through labour migration. The Keynesian policies pursued by larger and stronger economies were more difficult to sustain when the economic base was limited. In many situations, there was a shift towards the types of economic arrangements that prevailed in the pre-cash economy era; the involvement of the state in stepping up welfare was supplemented by civil society playing a bigger role.

Politically, comparisons can be drawn between the independent island states and the UK overseas territories. In the latter case, the British government had the ultimate responsibility, increasing support during COVID-19 but not without some tensions (e.g., in the British Virgin Islands). The independent island states did no worse given their circumstances. While one can point to the regional architecture that has developed in both the Caribbean and the Pacific islands region, the pandemic highlighted the limited agency of the island countries, buffeted as they were by developments occurring elsewhere.

Lessons to be learnt

A major lesson to be learnt from the experience of the Commonwealth countries in responding to the pandemic during 2020 is the crucial importance of political leadership. Moving early and decisively to deal with the pandemic required considerable political judgement, courage, critical assessment of emerging scientific evidence, and the ability to marshal political support. 'He who hesitates is lost' as the saying goes, and unfortunately 'lost' could be an understatement during the pandemic. On the other hand, one might counter with 'fools rush in where angels fear to tread'. Leaders needed to be both decisive and wise, taking heed of and balancing between the best scientific and economic advice.

Having strong measures designed to suppress the virus as soon as possible seemed to be the most effective strategy. This might have caused a severe economic downturn in the first instance, but if a large measure of suppression were achieved, then one could be on the road to economic recovery earlier than would otherwise be the case. Strong Keynesian measures were generally the preferred economic instrument for ensuring economic survival; whether centre-right governments would continue with this approach remained to be seen.

While governments generally focused on national interests as they saw them, it was not entirely 'dog eats dog'. Some elements of international cooperation remained, as with the multilateral, WHO-spearheaded COVAX facility, enabling developed countries to assist developing countries in obtaining a COVID-19 vaccine. Most countries involved in development assistance adapted their programmes to provide support relating to the pandemic.

This is where the Commonwealth has a role, whether acting through the Commonwealth Secretariat or a forum such as CHOGM (previously due to meet in Kigali, Rwanda, June 2021, but postponed to June 2022). The Secretariat acted as an information clearinghouse for programmes relating to COVID-19, but perhaps more important was the role of the Commonwealth in promoting and upholding norms of international cooperation. As a grouping covering such a wide range of states, there is scope to try out and build support for proposals before putting them in more universal contexts, such as different United Nations bodies, including the WHO. For example, one suggestion for Kigali 2021 (now Kigali 2022) was that CHOGM should promote the goal of a 'cleaner, greener recovery', linking climate change to post-COVID-19 concerns (Ransome, 2020). Another proposal was that the Commonwealth, along with other relevant bodies, should promote international cooperation to prepare for future pandemics and to facilitate vaccine development and distribution (Doherty, 2021).

Acknowledgement

Professor David Dunt (Melbourne School of Population and Global Health (MSPGH), University of Melbourne) provided helpful feedback on an earlier version of the Introduction.

Note

1 The statistics on COVID-19 assume accurate record keeping in the various countries covered; this is not necessarily the case in some instances.

References

Doherty, P. (2021). COVID-19 and beyond. *The Round Table: The Commonwealth Journal of International Affairs*, 110 (1), 171–172, https://doi.org/10.1080/00358533.2021.1875717

Ransome, D. (2020, 11 September). The Commonwealth: Towards Kigali 2021, Commonwealth Round Table, www.commonwealthroundtable.co.uk/general/health/covid-19/the-commonwealth-towards-kigali-2021/

Triggle, N. (2020, 17 December). Covid vaccine: More than 130,000 vaccinated in UK in first week. BBC News, www.bbc.com/news/health-55332242

In, but not of, Africa: a divided South Africa faces COVID-19

Steven Friedman

ABSTRACT
A feature of the COVID-19 pandemic has been that many 'First World' countries have been less able to prevent illnesses and deaths than some in the 'Third World'. But what if a country is both 'First' and 'Third' World? This article argues that South Africa is such a country and that its response to COVID-19 has been shaped by this reality. That explains why the African country with the most sophisticated health facilities on the continent has experienced almost as many cases and fatalities as the rest of Africa combined.

Introduction

IF one country is more like two countries, it is bound to find it difficult to come to terms with a common peril.

On two levels, South Africa's response to COVID-19 has been unlike any other in Africa. First, its seeming sophistication is unique on the continent. It quickly embraced the familiar mantra 'following the science'; as in some countries outside the continent, medical scientists have advised the government and have become media celebrities. The public has been regaled with statistical models predicting case and fatality numbers. The government adopted a 'risk adjusted' strategy in which five levels of lockdown, of varying severity, could be imposed, regionally or on the entire country. Second, South Africa has experienced almost as many cases and fatalities as the rest of Africa combined (BBC News, 2020).Why did the country with the most sophisticated medical infrastructure on the continent experience by far the most severe outbreak? This may well have happened because of, not despite, its sophistication, or because of realities of which the sophistication is a symptom.

Around the world, COVID-19 has challenged the familiar distinction between the 'First World' with its 'developed' economy, infrastructure and institutions and the 'Third World' which is assumed to lag far behind. More than a few 'First World' countries – the United States and United Kingdom chief among them – experienced far more recorded cases and deaths (in total and as a ratio of population) than 'Third World' countries such as Vietnam and Rwanda (Johns Hopkins University Coronavirus Resource Centre [JHU], 2020). While it may be years before we fully understand why COVID-19 did far more damage in some parts of the world than others, one plausible hypothesis is that 'First World' countries are leaders in curative medicine, which is of limited value against a virus for which there is no cure. Pandemics require a public health response; parts of the 'Third World' are better equipped because they are used to threats to public health. As in East Asian countries which have faced several coronavirus outbreaks, in parts of Africa, epidemics such as Ebola required responses not unlike that required by COVID-19.

But what if a country is both 'First World' and 'Third World'? South Africa is such a country. Its economy and social infrastructure were built to serve the needs of a white minority which believed itself to be a small sliver of Western Europe and North America on the dark continent. While a quarter century of democracy has brought important changes, the patterns which underpinned minority rule have largely survived. A minority of 'insiders', no longer all white, live much as Britons or Americans do. The 'outsider' majority, still almost entirely black, live much like the poor in other 'Third World' countries. The difference between their realities lies deeper than the fact that some are much richer than others – that is true today of just about every society (Piketty, 2014). The two really are, in a sense, different worlds. The assumptions which underpin life in the one differ fundamentally to those on which the other rests.

This article argues that South Africa's response to COVID-19 has reflected this reality. First, the society's realities made it more susceptible than its neighbours: the first reported case was that of a couple returning from a holiday in Italy (National Institute for Communicable Diseases [NICD], 2020), an option not available to almost all citizens of other African countries. Second, the government and its scientific advisors assumed from the outset that the virus could be managed but not eliminated or effectively contained. This approach was built on a reading of the European and American experience. It also assumed that most citizens – those who inhabit the 'Third World' – were incapable of protecting themselves in the manner required and would do so only if they were coerced. Since this fundamentally misread the reality, it reduced the country's capacity to prevent a widespread outbreak and ensured outcomes far worse than those in the rest of the continent.

'Following the science'

Like governments elsewhere in the world, South Africa's has insisted throughout that it is 'following the science' (Machanik, 2020). This had a special significance in the light of a chapter in the country's recent history.

The previous epidemic which it faced, HIV and AIDS, was worsened, during the tenure of the country's second President elected by universal franchise, Thabo Mbeki, by government hostility to the prevailing scientific consensus and the medical scientists who advocated it. Mbeki, probably because he was reacting against attitudes which portrayed AIDS as a disease spread by the sexual habits of black people, (Friedman, 2010) became an AIDS denialist: the only scientists to whom he gave a sympathetic hearing were a small group of dissidents whose claims were discredited by the scientific mainstream. Activists campaigning for affordable treatment for people living with AIDS (which Mbeki and his government resisted) made much of the 'marginalisation' of the scientists: Mbeki's attitude was compared to Lysenkoism, the elevation by Stalin of the theories of the pseudo-scientist Lysenko to state doctrine which was beyond question (Geffen, 2005).

The government's response to COVID-19 was the polar opposite. It established a Medical Advisory Council, chaired by Salim Abdool Karim, one of the scientists who

Mbeki rejected, and including some others who suffered similar treatment. It made much of its partnership with scientists, some of whom it afforded platforms to inform the country of current scientific evidence on COVID-19. The government's response was led by the minister of health, Zweli Mkhize, a medical doctor who was a classmate of Karim's at medical school. Activists and journalists, as well as Karim himself, marvelled at the contrast between this response and Mbeki's stance on AIDS (Du Plessis, 2020). The government response was also compared favourably to that of the US and Brazilian governments, which were founded on a denial of the importance of COVID-19 and the need to compromise the economy to fight it.

COVID-19 arrived in South Africa early in March. Over the first two weeks, it spread exponentially: Karim noted that it followed the pattern of the United Kingdom and other severely affected countries (Africa News Agency [ANA], 2020). This pattern was initially halted by the first significant government response, in late March – a severe lockdown. President Cyril Ramaphosa underlined the government's enthusiasm for science by announcing that this decision was a product of its 'risk adjusted strategy' to COVID-19 (Ramaphosa, 2020). He promised that the government would use extensive screening and testing to identify people who had contracted COVID-19. (Brandt, 2020). The scientific language contrasted sharply with AIDS denialism and elicited much admiration for the government's respect for science. This time, it seemed, it was guided by knowledge, not politics.

But the comforting image of an effective partnership between government and science ignored uncomfortable realities. The parallel between AIDS and COVID-19 was not as clear as the parallel suggested. When AIDS became contentious in South Africa (from the early 2000s to Mbeki's resignation in 2008), the science was clear. There was consensus on what caused the virus's spread and what should be done about it – medicine was available which reduced it to a chronic condition and enabled infected people to live a normal life. For much of the controversy over HIV and AIDS, the demand that the government listen to scientists boiled down to the insistence that it recognise that anti-retroviral drugs can treat HIV positive people effectively and make them available to infected people. COVID-19 is a new illness and the science is evolving. To name but one example, in the early stages of the pandemic it was assumed that only droplets on surfaces spread the infection – later, evidence suggested that it was airborne, which required different preventive strategies (Pijoos, 2020). There is still no scientific consensus on many aspects of COVID-19 and how to fight it.

'Following the science' was, therefore, not a straightforward – and self-evidently beneficial – choice because it begged the question of which science to follow. As some heated arguments between South African scientists (and between rival views in the United Kingdom) showed, there are competing 'sciences' (Lehulere, 2020). If policy-makers simply leave the choice to the scientists they have chosen to trust, 'following the science' still means choosing a strategy which will inevitably be rejected by some credible scientists. In South Africa, this became evident in a way which went unnoticed by the national debate but may partly explain why it suffered so many more illnesses and deaths than its neighbours.

While South African medical scientists disagreed loudly on some issues, they (or at least all of them whose view was heard by the lay public), agreed on one point which was presented to the society as an expression of 'the science' – despite the fact that it differed from the view of many mainstream scientists in other parts of the world. In his first public statements on COVID-19, Karim, by then installed as chair of the Medical Advisory Council, declared that it was 'inevitable that South Africa will experience a severe epidemic' because 'the rest of the world' had been unable to avoid it and the country was no different from the rest of the planet (Matiwane & Muller, 2020). The purpose of preventive measures – the recently imposed lockdown – was not to prevent mass infections but to 'buy time' by ensuring that the health system could cope with the cases it would inevitably be required to treat.

This view was never challenged in South Africa's usually noisy and polarised public debate. The media, interest groups, citizens' organisations and political parties accepted it without question. But the claim that all countries were experiencing a severe epidemic was untrue. African countries had, at the time Karim spoke, experienced few cases, which immediately contradicted the claim that all countries had experienced a severe epidemic. Some countries and territories – much of East Asia, New Zealand and the Indian state of Kerala were then much-reported examples – had experienced rising case numbers but had, at the time, contained them, limiting cases and deaths. (JHU, 2020) Why did Karim, a scientist with an international reputation, base his prediction on a claim so out of kilter with the information available to any newspaper reader? Why did he present it as a scientific truism when he must have known that, at precisely that time, colleagues elsewhere were arguing (as they still do) that the task of preventative measures should be to 'crunch the curve', not simply to flatten it (Sridhar, 2020) which means stopping the spread of the virus to prevent a severe epidemic, rather than delaying its spread to ready the health system? Why was this view endorsed by his South African colleagues? Why did just about no-one challenge it?

The stress on readying the health system was also never challenged. While this was regarded as 'common sense', it isn't as obvious as it seems. Because there is no cure for COVID-19 and, in March, there were no proven effective treatments, it could not be assumed that patients would recover if they were able to access the system. The treatments which were assumed at the outset to be essential – placing very ill patients on ventilators – appear to have been relatively ineffective and medical opinion later came to favour less invasive treatments (Begley, 2020). So, it was not self-evident at the time that readying the health system would help patients to recover and even less evident that this was a superior option to trying to prevent a severe outbreak. But at no stage during the epidemic have the interests and institutions who are meant to hold the government to account (and often do so very loudly) pressed it to say how effective treatment has been. The key question, whether using the health system enabled patients who would have otherwise died to recover, was never asked. When academics raised the issue in public, they were ignored (Machanik, 2020). Why was the strategy centred around the health system given these realities? And why did no-one with any influence in the public debate ask whether it made more sense to ready the health system than to try to so contain the virus that few people would fall ill?

We will return to these questions. First, it is necessary to describe how the severe epidemic occurred, not because it was unavoidable but because government strategy made it so.

Soft underbelly

South Africa's lockdown, which began on March 27, three weeks after the first case had been reported, was particularly severe.

It began at Level 5, the most stringent. It imposed bans on movement adopted by other countries, closing all business premises except those of 'essential services'. No movement outside homes was allowed unless the people moving were essential workers or could show they were on their way to buy necessities or seeking medical help. This meant, of course, that no exercise outside private homes was permitted. Unusually, it banned the sale of tobacco products and alcohol; food stores were forbidden to sell cooked food. Some 73 000 troops were deployed on the streets to help police enforce the rules (Daniel, 2020).

While the initial public response was supportive, middle-class and affluent suburban residents soon began to complain about the restrictions. When the government began easing them, middle-class resistance became particularly vocal after Ramaphosa announced that cigarette sales would be permitted only to backtrack after Nkosazana Dlamini Zuma, the Cabinet minister whose department was responsible for imposing the rules (and who happened to have campaigned against smoking since she served as health minister), insisted that 'public opinion' (which she had manufactured by encouraging anti-smoking groups to complain) was opposed to tobacco and cigarette sales. (Mahlakoana, 2020) Anger was mixed with ridicule when the government allowed the sale of winter clothing but published regulations specifying in comic detail which items could be sold (Tjiya, 2020). Ironically, there is evidence that clothing retailers played a major role in writing the maligned rules, but this was never reported.[1]

Shortly after the lockdown began, organised business, which first endorsed the measures, began lobbying furiously for their easing. Later, religious organisations began pressing to resume services. Soon, businesses in every sector of the economy, including travel and tourism (which would seem to be most dangerous in a pandemic) and organisations responsible for every other form of human activity were insisting that they were essential to national well-being. If the government was 'following the science', this lobbying would have been ignored since scientific advice counselled against opening activity when infection levels are rising. But, amid rising case numbers, the government began relaxing restrictions.

It was forced to do this because it failed to use the lockdown to stop the virus in its tracks. Other countries could ease restrictions as infection rates were dropping for one of two reasons. Either they locked down late, after the epidemic had grown exponentially – restrictions or the trajectory of the virus or both ensured a drop in rates. Or they had used the lockdown to implement effective testing and tracing: their lockdowns reduced case numbers enough to make testing all infected people and tracing all their contacts a realistic possibility. South Africa locked down early and did indicate that testing and tracing was the next step in the process. But, although the government has continued to publish figures showing that millions of people have been tested, testing does not help to control COVID-19's spread unless results are available rapidly (since contacts must be traced quickly). Yet tests soon began to back up at the national laboratory (Low, 2020) and this ensured that, even if tracing had been effective – and there was evidence that in parts of the country with rising infection rates it was not – the backlog in the laboratory meant that test results would not be available in time to trace contacts.

This ensured that, despite the lockdown, infections were rising when the suburban middle class was venting about the restrictions and business and other lobbies were pressing for their end. It is one of the great ironies of South Africa's battle against COVID-19 that the Achilles heel was not, as was widely assumed, people living in poverty in high density townships or shack settlements but a high-tech pathology lab. (Almost immediately after the lockdown began, a range of voices argued that, while it had a good chance of achieving its aim in the suburbs, its prospects were much slimmer in the places where most people live).

Official data suggests that, despite these constraints, the restrictions were relatively effective at controlling the spread (Derived from Makgetla & Maiwashe, 2020). During the two most stringent lockdown periods, only two of nine provinces experienced severe outbreaks: one was the Western Cape, the only province in which the black African poor are not in a majority. In the other seven, including Gauteng, the country's economic hub, levels rose but were contained. Karim marvelled that infections had slowed so markedly that 'we have a different trajectory than we have seen anywhere else in the world' (ANA, 2020).

The fact that Western Cape was worst affected was important politically because it is the only province controlled by an opposition party – the Democratic Alliance, a party primarily of the affluent suburbs. Much media opinion, which tends to be hostile to the governing African National Congress, and sees suburbs as fonts of efficiency, insisted that greater testing was the reason. But hospital admissions and deaths in the province were also substantially higher, showing that testing was not the reason (ANA, 2020a): the province's premier was the first to complain that test results were backed up, which weakens the claim that its testing was identifying outbreaks which other provinces were missing. While it is still not clear whether Western Cape was initially the epicentre because its response was lacking or because it happens to be more exposed to tourism, South Africa's deep political divisions ensured that no serious attempt was made to answer this question.

Later, infections, hospital admissions and deaths in the other provinces began rising sharply – but only when restrictions were significantly eased at the beginning of June to allow parts of the economy to open (derived from Makgetla & Maiwashe, 2020). This suggests strongly that it was the failure of testing and tracing which was the soft underbelly of the government campaign, not the constraints and habits of the urban poor. During June and July, the country experienced a surge in infections which, by early August, was equivalent in cases per 100 000 people, to numbers in the United States and some Latin American countries (Makgetla & Maiwashe, 2020). Case numbers began to subside in August and, by the end of the month, had reached a plateau. Between late August and mid-November, daily case numbers and fatalities remained steady – on average there were 1 656 new infections and 84 deaths each day.[2] Cases were not spread evenly through the country and are usually a consequence of 'cluster outbreaks' in particular regions – only two provinces accounted for the bulk of the increase (Business Tech, 2020).

Trends since August convinced much of the national debate that the virus had been effectively contained, although concerns about a 'second wave' persisted. But the South African debate's notion of an acceptable level of daily infections and deaths is several times higher than the rate which, in several other countries, is considered serious enough to warrant emergency measures – in mid-November, South Korea warned of an impending crisis because it reported around 200 daily cases for several days. (Shin, 2020) This, with the already mentioned reality that cases and deaths remained steady at around half those in the entire African continent, questioned the mainstream consensus that the country had done well at containing the virus.

One state, two countries

To make sense of these realities, we need to understand some core features of contemporary South Africa.

If official data is to be believed, South Africa is the most unequal country in the world (Beaubien, 2018). This has important implications for its fight against COVID-19. It is hardly the only country in the world where some live in comfortable suburbs, many others in under-serviced slums. What makes South Africa highly unusual in Africa – and far more like a Latin American country – is that it is divided not only into rich and poor but into two very different worlds. It may, therefore, be no accident that Latin America has experienced high levels of COVID-19 cases and deaths (JHU, 2020) and that, while South Africa has not experienced the overwhelmed health systems and massed burials which plagued much of Latin America, its experience in relation to the rest of the continent is much like Latin America's in relation to the rest of the world.

Before 1994, South Africa was a legally enforced racial oligarchy, the product of Dutch and British colonisation. The country became a republic in 1960, but the structure of the society and the culture which underpins it have important colonial features. White rule sought to transplant the culture of Europe and North America into Africa: whites tend to see those parts of the world as exemplars (even when they complained during apartheid that their governments were insufficiently supportive of white rule) and they sought to build infrastructure and institutions modelled on those of 'the West'. Visitors during this period would note that the whites-only suburbs of the major cities resembled southern California. Like the citizens of those societies, whites enjoyed the vote and civil liberties provided they did not identify overly with black demands.

The black majority was excluded from this world except as providers of menial labour. It was, therefore, common for critics of white rule to remark on the stark contrast between affluent white suburbs with their 'First World' amenities and poverty-stricken, under-served areas where the majority lived which were much the same as similar areas elsewhere in Africa, Latin America and Asia. Black people were denied either the vote or civil liberties (Dingake, 1987).

The end of white rule in 1994 might have been expected to produce a decisive move away from these divisions towards a culture and institutions which met the needs of all citizens. It did not. One possible consequence of a social reality in which one group enjoys amenities, rights and privileges by dominating another is that the way of life of the dominant group may come to be seen as the norm: the privileges of the dominant may come to define the 'good society' and any diminution of that standard might be seen as an expectation that the formerly dominated should make do with less than the minority enjoyed when it dominated. This is what happened in South Africa and it has defined the first quarter century of democracy.

For the elite which took over government in 1994 (and much of the intelligentsia and professional class which grew in size and influence after democracy was achieved), the unstated goal of the new society came to be the extension to all that which the white minority enjoyed under apartheid (Friedman, in press). In a society still deeply divided by race, this is one assumption which tacitly unites the new black elite and the old white one, whose lifestyle is still the desired norm, now blessed with the sanction of democratic legitimacy. This does not mean that nothing has changed since 1994: a great deal has. But the consensus has ensured a development path devoted to squeezing as many black people as possible into the institutions of suburban society (including the upper echelons of the economy) rather than fundamentally changing them. Since it is not possible to extend to most or all what a small minority enjoyed by using force to dominate the vast majority, a core feature of apartheid, a division of society into insiders who enjoy the benefits of the market economy and outsiders who do not, remains – albeit with the inclusion of a significant minority of black people in the insider group. And, while there has been constant talk since 1994 of reorienting the country's international partnerships away from North America and Europe, its elite continues to see the global North as the centre of gravity, even when its example is seen as one to avoid.

One further consequence is that the lives and experiences of the majority, a stark reminder that much of the country does not enjoy the 'First World' lifestyle which the elite sees as the desired norm, are seen as an embarrassment. Poverty is an appropriate source of shame. But it those who live in it who cause embarrassment, not the condition. One of the more enduring fantasies of post-1994 South Africa is that, despite the decline of traditional jobs throughout the world, it will somehow be possible to revive the days when all whites were employed in formal work and extend that to everyone. Informal economic activity is thus seen as an 'indecent' job, even if it generates wealth and those who engage in it show great ingenuity (African National Congress [ANC], 2019).

This context illustrates why South Africa is not simply a country in which some do very well and many are poor: it is also one whose history has ensured that it is the only country in Africa where two very different social and economic worlds cohabit. Since the dominant groups live in and value the "First World' features of the major cities, it is their view which is imposed on the majority living in a very different world (although there are important points of intersection).

In the South looking North

Armed with this background, we can begin to make sense of a reaction to COVID-19 which may have made high case and fatality numbers (at least by African standards) almost inevitable.

The root of the problem is the scientific consensus that a severe epidemic was inevitable, backed by the inaccurate claim that no country had avoided one by March, 2020. The questions posed earlier about this can be answered by pointing to two related probabilities. The first is that, when the scientific establishment concluded that no country had escaped one, they meant that no country which is important to them had done this. The dominant world view does not look for international trends in South Korea, New Zealand or Rwanda. It looks to the United States and Western Europe, which did not avoid a severe epidemic (some more peripheral European countries such as Greece and Portugal initially did but they are generally not what the mainstream has in mind when it thinks of Europe). (My Broadband, 2020)

It was common at the early stages of the pandemic for the government and those close to it to warn that South Africa should avoid becoming like Italy, the US, Spain and the UK. No one suggested that it should seek to emulate South Korea or Rwanda; not even China earned a positive mention despite the fact that South Africa courts Chinese investment and its membership of the BRICS alliance makes it a development partner. Not once since the epidemic began have the responses of African or Asian countries been the subject of mainstream discussion. The scientific mainstream's perspective was encapsulated in an interview Karim gave to *Nature*, in which he acknowledged that hospitalisations and deaths were low in 'Africa' but added: 'I don't have the answer … At the moment, it's an enigma. The reason will reveal itself in due course' (Nordling, 2020). In an interview with the BBC he confessed to being 'all at sea' as he tried to make sense of this (Harding, 2020).

Karim's candour is refreshing (and unusual among South African scientists) but revealing. Like many of his colleagues, the government's chief advisor refers to Africa as a distant and exotic terrain, despite the fact that a twist of fate made the country's president chair of the African Union for 2020. Also, the stock response of an epidemiologist puzzled by the progression of an epidemic in other countries would surely be to consult colleagues there. This idea seems not to have occurred to him despite the fact that he chairs the UNAIDS Scientific Expert Panel and belongs to World Health Organisation committees. Revealingly, he also belongs to the US National Academy of Medicine, the American Academy of Microbiology and the Association of American Physicians. (SAMRC, n.d). This international scientific figure apparently either knows of no colleague elsewhere on the continent or does not believe those he does know worth consulting. There is nothing in these responses to distinguish the speaker from an American or European scientist musing on the latest mystery to emerge from 'the dark continent'

It is safe to assume that when Karim said a severe epidemic was inevitable, he knew that some countries had avoided this fate. So, surely, did his colleagues who disagreed with him on other issues but not this one. It seems likely, therefore, that what they were really assuming (and did not say because it might be impolitic) was that a severe epidemic was inevitable not everywhere but in South Africa. They may have believed this either because they felt the health system was inadequate or that it would be difficult to enforce public health measures in the country's 'Third World' areas. Both display 'First World' biases.

On misgivings about the health system, it was noted earlier that limiting COVID-19's harm depends on public health measures. If the scientists were worried about health capabilities, they do seem to have been assuming, as their colleagues in the 'First World' did, that curative medicine was a key to fighting COVID-19. This would explain the stress on readying the health system despite the lack of certainty, particularly in the early stages of the epidemic, that curative medicine would assist patients. That neither the government nor the scientists were ever asked by the media or citizens' groups to say whether hospitals were assisting COVID-19 patients may similarly be explained by the assumption by all of 'First World' South Africa that all human ills are cured by curative medicine.

The assumption, mentioned earlier, that people living in poverty may be unable to protect themselves is not necessarily a symptom of bias. Many in 'Third World' South Africa lack access to clean water to wash their hands and live in overcrowded conditions which make physical distancing difficult (Garba, 2020); minibus taxis, the dominant mode of transport for people living in poverty, are sources of danger since they usually pack in many passengers and are poorly ventilated, but they are often the only means of transport for people needing to reach their work places. The medical scientists' public interventions rarely if ever stressed the need to provide washing stations for people lacking water or suggestions for protecting people in overcrowded homes. Some did tell journalists that overcrowding in taxis was a health hazard, but only so that they could denounce lockdown measures (News 24 Wire, 2020). And so, it seems likely that the assumption was based less on a recognition of the conditions of people living in poverty than the belief that only people in the suburbs were sophisticated and responsible enough to take the measures necessary to protect themselves.

This was clearly a government assumption, made ironic by the fact that 'Third World' citizens are the voters who keep the governing party in office. Dlamini Zuma partly justified the tobacco ban by warning that 'our people', code for poor, black, people, tended to share cigarettes (Jacobs, 2020). A cabinet colleague justified the ban on cooked food by warning that people in low income areas bought cooked meat from roadside stalls; (Modise, 2020) a ban on alcohol sales was said to prevent people engaging in drunken violence and so overburdening the health system (Head, 2020). A rule banning outdoor exercise after 9 a.m. was justified as an attempt to prevent people wandering in public (Davis, 2020). While it was these rules which triggered suburban anger, it is safe to assume that their purpose was not to prevent suburbanites smoking on porches, sipping cocktails, ordering sushi or walking dogs. It was to prevent assumed outbreaks of irresponsibility among the poor.

Empirical data on how well-founded these claims were is not available. Alcohol does fuel violence, largely in low income areas, which does place pressure in hospitals. But the assumption that people living in poverty are ignorant or irresponsible is dubious. Broadcast media coverage of township areas revealed that many people wore masks and often complained that they were being forced to queue for groceries (or food parcels) in circumstances which made distancing difficult. The (American) authors of a study on township attitudes to the virus found that people were so worried about their physical health that they insisted that restrictions would not impair their mental health – and then scolded them for their ignorance of mental health! (Mendenhall & Kim, 2020). There is copious evidence of deep-seated fears of riding in taxis (Mthethwa, 2020). When schools reopened, many of the people who were assumed not to know or care about COVID-19 were reluctant to send their children back to the classroom for fear of contracting the virus.(Ndlazi, 2020). Indeed, they may well have been more concerned to protect themselves than suburban residents who flocked back to restaurants when infection levels remained reasonably high.

Given this, had the government sought to build a partnership with people outside the suburbs to fight the virus, it might well have significantly reduced infections and fatalities. But this option was never attempted – instead, troops were deployed to enforce the regulations, often in a manner which violated the rights and in some cases cost the lives of citizens. This might have been avoided had 'First World' South Africans not assumed that their 'Third World' compatriots were unable and unwilling to protect themselves against COVID-19. The government claimed it relied on a network of citizen volunteers and also worked with community groups to distribute food relief to citizens (Zulu, 2020). But the volunteers and community groups were carrying out government decisions, not helping to make them. There is no evidence of any attempt to treat citizens' organisations as partners in designing a response to the virus.

The nature of South African society may also explain the peculiar nature of public debate on COVID-19. While other countries debated the efficacy of measures, South Africa did not – despite the fact that loudly denouncing government actions is one of the debate's staples. Not only was the claim that a severe epidemic was inevitable never challenged. When media reports revealed that test results were being delayed in the national laboratory, there was no reaction. To this author's knowledge, no journalist has asked either the government or its scientific advisors a single critical question on the medical or scientific aspect of the handling of the pandemic. The modelling exercises were also treated with reverence although they appear to be based on a 100-year-old model which may not understand the workings of the virus which causes COVID-19 (Gering & Ralekhetho, 2020). Instead, debate was devoted to an acrimonious shouting match between supporters and opponents of the lockdown. So all-consuming was this that any contribution to debate on COVID-19 was construed as support for or opposition to the lockdown and greeted with vitriol or adulation even when it clearly was neither.

It seems highly likely that the burden of serious COVID-19 cases and deaths fell largely on the 'Third World' section of society. This is based not on data – the government has refused to break down its statistics in any way which would enable identification of the groups most affected because it argues that this would stigmatise those whose numbers were high. It stems, rather, from the reality that debate in South Africa is monopolised by its 'First World' and expresses its concerns only. There was no great debate on how effective the fight against the virus was because, in the main, it was not 'First World' South Africa's problem. But the restrictions did affect it. After initially endorsing them, possibly because they felt that the suburbs did face a significant threat, 'First World' interests became increasingly irate. The lockdown debate was predictable, given 'First World' citizens' antipathy to the government which tends to unite whites and the black middle-class even though they are deeply divided on racial issues. The scientists who were hailed for opposing the lockdown seemed to be reflecting and amplifying suburban biases rather than making plausible scientific arguments – one very senior scientist was forced to retract a clearly inaccurate statement that a Johannesburg hospital which serves low-income townships had treated no malnutrition cases until the lockdown. Since they shared the biases of the anti-lockdown lobby, which enjoyed the support of organised business and the media, they were feted, not challenge (Heywood, 2020).

The veneration of scientists (which so afflicts some broadcast journalists that they sound deeply apologetic that they are forced to ask scientists even fawning questions) is also explained by these realities. Science is associated with 'First World' competence and those who practise it are therefore assumed to be bearers of civilisation's fruits. It is this which sets 'First World' South Africa apart from right-wingers around the world who denounce the wearing of masks and other measures to contain the virus even though the two share an antipathy to restrictions. Ironically, this may have shielded the government from criticism of its anti-COVID-19 measures even as it was pilloried for imposing restrictions on the suburbs. By 'following the science' the government which, despite its 'First World' perspective is identified with the 'Third World' by its many 'First World' detractors, was bowing to the superior ways of the 'First World'. The restrictions meant that 'Third World' politicians were ordering about their superiors, an assumption which has its roots in deeply embedded white supremacy (the government is overwhelmingly black, the suburbs mostly white) although some in the new black middle-class have complicated this diagnosis by adopting similar attitudes.

Finally, the fact that the government allowed lobbies to dictate the pace at which restrictions were eased also set it apart from the rest of the continent in which, while there were citizen demonstrations against lockdown rules, sustained lobbying for relaxations seemed less evident. While lobbies are not a purely 'First World' phenomenon, far more was at play here than the standard attempt by interest groups to influence policy. The lobbying was backed by an almost monolithic campaign in which media constantly stressed the distress of not only companies but anyone whose activities were restricted by government measures and reduced thousands of deaths and illnesses to a footnote (South Africans never saw on their television screens the pictures of hospital staff battling to treat ill people which citizens of many other countries saw). At the same time, the economic hardships of the majority were regularly invoked to support the political purpose of 'First World' lobbies – a phenomenon which is standard in South African debates in which the poor never speak but are constantly spoken about to serve agendas for which they are useful props. This orchestrated campaign, in which a range of private interests with a common agenda combine to create a particular 'common sense' view of what must be done is surely more likely in a society in which 'the First World' is used to shaping reality in its own image. Its effect was to significantly increase case and deaths as restrictions were removed not because testing and tracing was working but because the 'First World' demanded this.

South Africa's hybrid nature was responsible not only for its choice of strategy but also for the fact that its essentials were never challenged. It ensured that the battle against COVID-19 was declared lost before it began and that this set in motion events which made this prediction self-fulfilling. The result was what it always is in a society with South Africa's features: heightened suffering among its 'Third World' citizens caused by the concerns of the dominant 'First World' whose gaze fails to notice the damage it has caused.

Conclusion: the path not taken

What, if anything, could have been done to prevent this?

An effective response would have required a significant change of thinking among the elite, not only the politicians but scientists, media, academics, business people – all those whose decisions shape the society. Instead of seeing 'First World' strategies and technologies as the only appropriate tools, they could have given serious thought to ways of responding which recognised the realities facing most citizens and tailored responses to them – in a country with South Africa's profile there are ways of locating infected people and tracing their contacts which do not rely on a single laboratory using state-of-the-art methods. This would have entailed learning from the experiences of other countries in Africa and those in Asia rather than a tunnel vision which could see only Western Europe and North America.

More specifically, it was noted earlier that a partnership between the government and people living in poverty – residents of low-income townships and shack settlements – to tackle the virus was never attempted. Lest the proposal sound utopian, an example drawn from recent South African history indicates that it is not. South Africa boasts an extensive system of social grants, an effective anti-poverty instrument which distributes over 17 million grants (Motswai, 2018). The reach of the grants is largely the product of an initiative, begun in 1999, by Zola Skweyiya, the Minister responsible for grants, to extend their reach to everyone entitled to them. To this end, he instructed his public servants to reach out to all citizens' organisations in areas where people lived in poverty, asking them to identify anyone in their constituency who was entitled to a grant but did not get one (Amato, 2018). If partnering with citizens could extend social protection to millions, it could have offered them protection from a virus too.

In sum, a response was needed which acknowledged that the key to fighting COVID-19 was recognising that the battle would be won and lost in the areas in which most South Africans live and that strategies needed to be tailored to capacities in those areas. This entailed recognising that the people who live in these areas are citizens with capacities, not problems. Experience elsewhere in Africa suggests that this approach would have reduced infections and deaths to a fraction of those which the country has had to endure.

Notes

1. This information was gleaned from off the record discussions with market analysts.
2. Author's calculations derived from Department of Health (2020).

Disclosure statement

No potential conflict of interest was reported by the author.

References

Africa News Agency (ANA). (2020, April 13). SA's Covid-19 infection plateau is unprecedented: Ministerial adviser. *Independent on Line*. https://www.iol.co.za/news/politics/sas-covid-19-infection-plateau-is-unprecedented-ministerial-adviser-46661184

Africa News Agency (ANA). (2020a, May 29). Cape Town's Covid-19 spike occurred in malls in last weeks of hard lockdown: Prof Karim. *Independent on Line*. https://www.iol.co.za/news/south-africa/western-cape/cape-towns-covid-19-spike-occurred-in-malls-in-last-weeks-of-hard-lockdown-prof-karim-48691940

African National Congress (ANC). (2019). *Myanc: More jobs, more decent jobs*. https://www.anc1912.org.za/myanc-more-jobs-more-decent-jobs-httpstcoj1hes0kftg

Amato, C. A.(2018, April 13). Obituary: A leader with backbone. *Mail and Guardian*. https://mg.co.za/article/2018-04-13-00-obituary-a-leader-with-backbone/

BBC News. (2020, October 12). *Coronavirus in Africa tracker*. https://www.bbc.co.uk/news/resources/idt-4a11d568-2716-41cf-a15e-7d15079548bc

Beaubien, J. (2018, April 2). *The country with the world's worst inequality is ....* https://www.npr.org/sections/goatsandsoda/2018/04/02/598864666/the-country-with-the-worlds-worst-inequality-is

Begley, S. (2020, April 21). New analysis recommends less reliance on ventilators to treat coronavirus patients. *Statnews*. https://www.statnews.com/2020/04/21/coronavirus-analysis-recommends-less-reliance-on-ventilators/

Brandt, K. (2020, March 31). Ramaphosa: Covid-19 screening drive will be intensive and far-reaching. *Eye Witness News*. https://ewn.co.za/2020/03/31/ramaphosa-covid-19-screening-drive-will-be-intensive-and-far-reaching

Business Tech. (2020, November 16). *How Covid-19 has shifted in South Africa over the last two weeks: Mkhize*. https://businesstech.co.za/news/trending/448619/how-covid-19-has-shifted-in-south-africa-over-the-last-two-weeks-mkhize/

Daniel, L. (2020, April 23). Ramaphosa's decision to deploy 73 000 soldiers questions lockdown's end. *The South African*, .https://www.thesouthafrican.com/news/does-ramaphosa-sandf-army-deployment-indicate-a-lockdown-extension/

Davis, R. (2020, May 14). Unpacking the rationality of South Africa's lockdown regulations. *Daily Maverick*. https://www.dailymaverick.co.za/article/2020-05-14-unpacking-the-rationality-of-south-africas-lockdown-regulations/

Department of Health. (2020). *Covid-19 online resource and news portal* https://sacoronavirus.co.za/

Dingake, M. (1987). *My fight against apartheid*. Kliptown Books.

Du Plessis, C.A.(2020, March 27). How South Africa's action on Covid-19 contrasts sharply with its response to AIDS. *The Guardian*. https://www.theguardian.com/global-development/2020/may/27/how-south-africas-action-on-covid-19-contrasts-sharply-with-its-response-to-aids-coronavirus

Friedman, S. (2010). Seeing ourselves as others see us: Racism, technique and the Mbeki administration. In D. Glaser (Ed.), *Mbeki and after: Reflections on the legacy of Thabo Mbeki* (pp. 163–186). Wits University Press.

Friedman, S. (in press). *The prison of the past: South African democracy and minority rule's legacy*. Wits University Press.

Garba, N. (2020, June 12). South Africa: COVID-19, the working class and the poor in South Africa. *All Africa*. https://allafrica.com/stories/202006120943.html

Geffen, N. (2005, March). *Echoes of Lysenko: State-sponsored pseudo-science in South Africa.* CSSR Working Paper No. 149 Cape Town, Centre for Social Science Research, Aids and Society Research Unit.

Gering, M., & Ralekhetho, M. (2020, October 8). Walking through the pandemic modelling, exponential growth and herd immunity maze. *Daily Maverick.* https://www.dailymaverick.co.za/opinionista/2020-10-08-walking-through-the-pandemic-modelling-exponential-growth-and-herd-immunity-maze/

Harding, A. (2020, September 3). Coronavirus in South Africa: Scientists explore surprise theory for low death rate. *BBC.com.* https://www.bbc.com/news/world-africa-53998374

Head, T. (2020, March 26). SA's alcohol ban explained: Why booze is barred during lockdown. *The South African.* https://www.thesouthafrican.com/news/why-alcohol-sale-banned-south-africa-during-lockdown/

Heywood, M. (2020, May 26). Malnutrition, health services and democracy: The responsibility to speak out. *Daily Maverick.* https://www.dailymaverick.co.za/article/2020-05-26-malnutrition-health-services-and-democracy-the-responsibility-to-speak-out/#:~:text=One%20of%20Gray%E2%80%99s%20%E2%80%98sins%E2%80%99%20was%20to%20have%20had,a%20result%20of%20the%20prolongation%20of%20the%20lockdown.

Jacobs, K. (2020). *Dlamini-Zuma explains reasons for tobacco ban.* https://www.capetownetc.com/news/dlamini-zuma-explains-reasons-for-tobacco-ban/

Johns Hopkins University Coronavirus Resource Centre (JHU). (2020). *Covid-19 dashboard.* https://coronavirus.jhu.edu/map.html

Lehulere, O. (2020, June 5). Scientists against science: The campaign to open "the economy" in the time of Covid-19. *Karibu.* https://karibu.org.za/scientists-against-science-the-campaign-to-open-the-economy-in-the-time-of-covid-19/

Low, M. (2020, May 8). SA doctors concerned about severe Covid-19 testing delays. *Daily Maverick.* https://www.dailymaverick.co.za/article/2020-05-08-sa-doctors-concerned-about-severe-covid-19-testing-delays/

Machanik, P. (2020, July 9). Covid-19: Free the evidence' *Mail and Guardian.* https://mg.co.za/coronavirus-essentials/2020-06-09-covid-19-free-the-evidence/

Mahlakoana, T. (2020, June 10). Dlamini Zuma's reasons for tobacco sales plan are "all over the place", court hears. *EyeWitness News.* https://ewn.co.za/2020/06/10/dlamini-zuma-s-reasons-for-tobacco-sales-ban-all-over-the-place-court-hears

Makgetla, N. with, & Lutendo Maiwashe. (2020). *TIPS tracker: The economy and the pandemic.* Tshwane, Trade and Industry Policy Strategies.

Matiwane, Z., & Muller, P. (2020, April 23). SA will have a severe epidemic: Prof Salim Abdool Karim' *Sowetan Live.* https://www.sowetanlive.co.za/news/south-africa/2020-04-23-listen-sa-will-have-a-severe-epidemic-prof-salim-abdool-karim/

Mendenhall, E., & Kim, A. W. (2020, October 8). People in Soweto told us about their fears in the first weeks of South Africa's lockdown. *The Conversation.* https://theconversation.com/people-in-soweto-told-us-about-their-fears-in-the-first-weeks-of-south-africas-lockdown-142325

Modise, K. (2020, April 21). Patel explains why cooked food can't be sold during lockdown. *EyeWitness News.* https://ewn.co.za/2020/04/21/patel-explains-why-hot-food-can-t-be-sold-during-lockdown

Motswai, N. (2018, February). SASSA Beneficiaries smiling all the way to the bank. Vuk'unzenzele, SA Government Communications (GCIS). https://www.vukuzenzele.gov.za/sassa-beneficiaries-smiling-all-way-bank

Mthethwa, C. A.(2020, March 17). South Africa: Coronavirus - commuters fear infection in overcrowded taxis. *Buses and Trains.* https://allafrica.com/stories/202003170127.html

My Broadband. (2020, April 14). *The worst is yet to come in South Africa.* https://mybroadband.co.za/news/trending/347639-the-worst-is-yet-to-come-in-south-africa.html

National Institute for Communicable Diseases (NICD). (2020, March 5). *First case of Coronavirus Covid-19 reported in South Africa.* https://www.nicd.ac.za/first-case-of-covid-19-coronavirus-reported-in-sa/

Ndlazi, S. (2020, April 29). Covid-19: Back-to-school fears mount. *Pretoria News.* https://www.iol.co.za/pretoria-news/covid-19-back-to-school-fears-mount-47325768

News 24 Wire. (2020, July 14). *Medical experts slam govt for banning booze but loading taxis.* https://citizen.co.za/news/covid-19/2320867/medical-experts-slam-govt-for-banning-booze-but-loading-taxis/

Nordling, L. (2020, July 24). Our epidemic could exceed a million cases' — South Africa's top coronavirus adviser. *Nature.*

Pijoos, I. (2020, July 9). How to protect yourself from airborne transmission of Covid-19. *Times Live.* https://www.timeslive.co.za/news/south-africa/2020-07-09-how-to-protect-yourself-from-airborne-transmission-of-covid-19/

Piketty, T. (2014). *Capital in the 21st century.* Harvard.

Ramaphosa, C. A.(2020, August 15). *South Africa's risk adjusted strategy to manage spread of Coronavirus Covid-19 South African government.* https://www.gov.za/speeches/president-cyril-ramaphosa-south-africa%E2%80%99s-risk-adjusted-strategy-manage-spread-coronavirus

SA Medical Research Council (SAMRC). (n.d) *Prof Salim Abdool Karim.* https://www.samrc.ac.za/people/prof-salim-abdool-karim

Shin, H. (2020, November 17). South Korea to tighten social distancing, warns of new COVID-19 crisis. *Reuters.* https://www.reuters.com/article/us-health-coronavirus-southkorea-idUSKBN27W32M

Sridhar, D. (2020, April 22). Crunching the coronavirus curve is better than flattening it, as New Zealand is showing. *The Guardian.* https://www.theguardian.com/commentisfree/2020/apr/22/flattening-curve-new-zealand-coronavirus

Tjiya, E. (2020, May 14). Minister Ebrahim Patel dictates to fashion police *Sowetan.* https://www.sowetanlive.co.za/entertainment/2020-05-14-minister-ebrahim-patel-dictates-to-fashion-police/

Zulu, L. (2020, April 29). *Remarks by the minister of social development, Ms Lindiwe Zulu, on COVID-19 economic and social measures that were announced by President Cyril Ramaphosa ....* South African Government, Department of Social Development. https://www.dsd.gov.za/index.php/21-latest-news/127-remarks-by-the-minister-of-social-development-ms-lindiwe-zulu-on-covid-19-economic-and-social-measures-that-were-announced-by-president-cyril-ramaphosa

Canada and COVID-19: the longer-term geopolitical implications

Kim Richard Nossal

ABSTRACT
This article explores the geopolitical implications of COVID-19 for Canada. It argues that the pandemic accelerated changes that were already underway as a result of the Trump presidency. It traces the spread of the virus in Canada and measures taken to control it. Canada's response was markedly different to that of the US and the geostrategic fissures have deepened. The pandemic has played a major role in transforming thinking about U.S./Canada relations. Canada is now much more alone in North America and the world.

Introduction

Given how disruptive the novel coronavirus disease (COVID-19) pandemic has been – and how global its reach has been – it is perhaps not surprising that there has been a burgeoning literature on the nature of world politics after the pandemic (Drezner, 2020). Much of the prognostication has been sceptical: Nye (2020) provides an illustrative cautionary analysis, arguing that 'it is still much too early to predict a geopolitical turning point' in global politics because the pandemic will not alter key structural realities that undergird contemporary great-power relations. Nye's scepticism, it might be noted, is widely shared, especially in the United States; a survey of American international relations (IR) scholars taken in May 2020 revealed that 54% of the 946 scholars who responded believed that the pandemic would not fundamentally alter the distribution of power in world politics (Jackson et al., 2020, p. 3).

In this article, I side-step the question about whether the pandemic will prove to be a geopolitical turning point for global politics more broadly. Instead, I explore the geopolitical implications of the COVID-19 pandemic for Canada, arguing that the pandemic accelerated a shift in Canada's geostrategic 'location' in global politics that was already underway as a result of the election of Donald J. Trump as president of the United States in 2016. While the pandemic may not turn out to be a turning point for global politics, for Canada it has already ushered in a new era.

While the administration of Joe Biden that took office in January 2021 is attempting to restore American global leadership, it is likely that the post-post-Cold War era will be marked by a continued slow dismantling of American pre-eminence in global politics – ushering in the kind of 'post-American world' that Fareed Zakaria foresaw a decade ago

(Zakaria, 2012). But Canada is already deeply implicated in the dramatic shifts precipitated by Trump during his first term. By the end of 2019, Canada was no longer in the same geostrategic position that it had been during much of the post-Cold War era, a location that had been marked by American leadership of a liberal international order in which multilateralism was widely embraced and great-power competition was not the central feature of international relations. Moreover, Canada's own response to COVID-19, markedly different to the American response, has deepened those geostrategic fissures.

COVID-19 in Canada

The disease unfolded in Canada in ways not dramatically different from other countries. After the World Health Organization (WHO) initiated its own emergency operations on 1 January, the Canadian government activated its Emergency Operations Centre on 15 January, but few extraordinary measures were taken until the first Canadian case was recorded on 25 January, when a Toronto man who had been in Wuhan tested positive. Even then, the optimism that was evident in most countries about the novel coronavirus was shared in Canada. After the first case was reported, Canada's chief public health officer, Theresa Tam, tweeted that 'there is no clear evidence that this virus is spread easily from person to person. The risk to Canadians remains low' (Tam, 2020); she also endorsed the WHO advice that travel bans were unnecessary. Canada refused to follow Australia or the United States in excluding travellers from China, arguing that it would be discriminatory. As the prime minister, Justin Trudeau, put it on 5 March, 'There is a lot of misinformation out there, there is a lot of knee-jerk reaction that isn't keeping people safe' (K. Harris, 2020). Instead, travellers arriving in Canada from Hubei were asked to self-isolate for two weeks.

This approach changed dramatically when Canada recorded its first death from COVID-19 on 9 March and after the WHO officially declared the outbreak a global pandemic on 11 March (WHO, 2020). The next day, it was announced that Trudeau's spouse, Sophie Grégoire, had tested positive for COVID-19, and the prime minister began a 14-day self-quarantine. On 13 March, from quarantine, Trudeau announced a series of steps, including the closure of parliament for five weeks, limiting international flights into Canada, banning cruise ships until 1 July, and encouraging social distancing (Cecco, 2020a).

Following the WHO declaration, provincial and territorial governments moved to ban large gatherings and to regulate other activities. In some provinces, schools that had closed for the traditional one-week March Break were kept closed. Most universities moved to on-line instruction. On 13 March, the premier of Québec, François Legault, declared an emergency, limiting gatherings and prompting Montréal to close arenas, pools and libraries (Authier, 2020). In Ontario, the premier, Doug Ford, declared an emergency on 17 March, ordering that restaurants, bars, theatres, schools and day care centres be closed (Davidson, 2020). However, no province or territory embraced the kind of hard lockdown that we saw in France or in Victoria in Australia.

In anticipation of the economic disruptions that cancellations and closures would produce, the federal government quickly put together a package of measures to cope with the disruption. The COVID-19 Economic Response Plan (CERP) was announced seven days after the WHO declaration. It included CAD$27 billion in direct support to workers and businesses; CAD$55 billion in tax deferrals to businesses and households; an increase in the Canada Child Benefit, a tax-free federal payment to eligible families with children; an increase in the credit on the Goods and Services Tax paid to low-incomes Canadians; an interest-free moratorium on Canada Student Loans owed by tertiary students; and a new Indigenous Community Support Fund for First Nations, Inuit and Métis Nation communities (Trudeau, 2020). Each of the provinces and territories introduced their own relief programmes for businesses and individuals. The federal government offered CAD $14 billion in June to provincial and territorial governments that were willing to agree to working with the federal government on 'safe restart' measures (Rabson, 2020). In April, to forestall large-scale layoffs, the federal government introduced the Canada Emergency Wage Subsidy programme, allowing employers to receive a 75% subsidy on wages retroactive to 15 March (Ibbitson, 2020).

The federal government also changed its policy on international travel. On 16 March, Trudeau announced that Canada would turn away all international visitors arriving by air with the exception of Americans, flight crews, and diplomats (Cecco, 2020b). The Canadian and U.S. governments announced the joint closure of their land border to all non-essential travel on 18 March. However, because Ottawa wanted to ensure the viability of the complex supply chains across the Canada-U.S. border, many of which depended on truck traffic through many of the 119 land border crossings that dot the border, truck drivers were exempted from quarantine requirements. However, because some 29,000 trucks cross the border every day, the border continued to be relatively porous throughout the pandemic.

When the federal government issued an advisory against travel outside Canada in March, a number of providers of travel health insurance immediately announced that medical coverage outside Canada would be suspended or restricted, prompting Trudeau to advise all Canadians abroad to return home (Tasker, 2020a). In the following week, more than a million Canadians and permanent residents made their way home (Jones, 2020), many of them families taking March Break vacations, but most of them 'snowbirds' (as those who spend harsh Canadian winters in warm American locations are called).

However, little effort was made to control this massive inflow. Instead returnees were given 'border tips' jointly issued by the Canadian Border Services Agency and the Canadian Snowbirds Association that did nothing more than ask them to self-isolate at home for 14 days (Canadian Border Services Agency, 2020). While the prime minister threatened to use the stiff penalties of the Quarantine Act, little was actually done. Needless to say, there were numerous reports of snowbirds returning to Canada not self-isolating.

While social distancing and hand sanitisation was put in place across Canada quickly, the other component of public health in the COVID-19 pandemic – masking – was slower to emerge. Because the WHO continued to insist well into May that there was not enough medical evidence for the benefits of mask-wearing, and because there was a persistent fear that a move to mask-wearing would deplete supplies of medical masks, the federal government was slow to embrace mask-wearing. While the federal airline regulator, Transport Canada, began to require masks for all air travellers in April, it was not until mid-May that Tam issued new regulations, replacing the 'suggestion' that everyone wear a mask with a 'recommendation' that masks be worn (Woods, 2020). However, it was largely left to municipalities to make mask-wearing mandatory via local by-laws, so that by the middle of the summer, mask-wearing in public places was widespread. Importantly, Trudeau himself promoted mask-wearing early on, even if the government he headed was hesitant. A mask, he said at a coronavirus briefing on 7 April, 'protects others more than it protects you … It prevents you from breathing or speaking moistly on them' (Elliott, 2020). While he immediately kicked himself for the phrase – 'What a terrible image,' he muttered to the cameras – it could be argued that the 'speaking moistly' gaffe actually helped ensure that in Canada mask-wearing was never politicised to the extent that it was in the United States (Van der Linden, 2020). While some Canadians tried to import anti-mask politics from the United States, the effort was both marginal and unsuccessful. A September public opinion poll, for example, showed that 83% of Canadians supported government mandates for mask-wearing at all indoor public spaces (Berthiaume, 2020).

Because Canada did not close down like Australia or New Zealand, but because Canadians and their political leaders generally took COVID-19 far more seriously than Americans and their leaders, the health impact of the pandemic was less severe than in the United States, but far more severe than in Australia, New Zealand and other 'successful' jurisdictions like South Korea, Taiwan and Hong Kong. By December 2020, Canada had over 385,000 cases, with 12,300 deaths (Canada, 2020). With a population of 37.8 million, the mortality rate was 325 deaths per million, well above the 35 deaths per million in Australia and 5 per million in New Zealand, but well below the 841 deaths per million in the United States (Worldometer, 2020).

The Canadian cases – and deaths – were not spread evenly across the country. As of December 2020, the north – Yukon, Northwest Territories, and Nunavut – have only had a tiny number of cases and just one death. The Atlantic provinces – Newfoundland and Labrador, Prince Edward Island, New Brunswick and Nova Scotia – took a hard-line approach to travel from other provinces, with the result that what is known in Canada as the 'Atlantic Bubble' suffered very few deaths: none in PEI, seven in New Brunswick, four in Newfoundland and Labrador, and 65 in Nova Scotia. Saskatchewan had 51 deaths and Manitoba 328. British Columbia had 457 and Alberta 551. The major centres of COVID-19 mortality have been Québec (7,084) and Ontario (3,663). In particular the cities of Toronto, Ottawa and Montréal struggled with renewed surge at the end of the summer and the reopening of schools, colleges, and universities; and, like many other countries, they experienced a very sharp spike in infections in October and November. Most of the deaths from COVID in Canada have been in long-term care facilities: when she delivered her annual report in October 2020, Teresa Tam, the Chief Public Health Officer, reported that fully 80% of COVID-19–related deaths occurred in long-term care facilities (Public Health Agency of Canada, 2020, p. 10, table 2), well above the average for Organisation for Economic Cooperation and Development (OECD) countries (Grant, 2020).

Because the United States is so central to Canadians, the differences in how the COVID-19 pandemic has affected each country played an important role in thinking about the future of the Canada-U.S. relationship. Mustapha and Van Rythoven (2020) put it well: Canadians watching the American response to COVID-19 'is more akin to watching a close friend spiral into a crisis of shockingly irresponsible behaviour. Not only is their tragic circumstance a threat to the safety of others, but we face the added grief of knowing that someone we care about has chosen such a destructive path.'

The geopolitical implications for Canada

Even before the COVID-19 pandemic broke out, Canada was finding itself in a radically different geostrategic position in global politics. There is considerable consensus among students of Canadian foreign policy on the factors that caused this disruption: the rise of great-power competition as a result of the growing assertiveness of the People's Republic of China under President Xi Jinping and the revanchism of the Russian Federation under Vladimir Putin; the rise of authoritarianism and right-wing populism; and the corrosive political effects of social media – these are commonly mentioned. However, there is one factor that all agree have radically altered Canadian foreign policy: the rise of Trump (see, inter alia, Boucher, 2020; Burney & Hampson, 2020; Greenhill & Welsh, 2020a, 2020b; Juneau, 2020; Mustapha & Van Rythoven, 2020; Paris, 2020).

The distal driver of this shift was the political transformation in the United States that would bring Trump to power. Simply put, 'American politics went insane,' to use Rauch's (2016) pithy but memorable explanation. Rauch traces the thirty-year process by which the American political system became increasingly dysfunctional as a result of growing hyper-partisanship. Trump's path to the White House in 2016 might have depended on just 77,744 votes in three battleground states, but it was that 'insanity,' Rauch argued, that made Trump, and Trumpism, possible. For Canada, however, that tiny number of votes dramatically transformed its geostrategic environment, for in power Trump radically challenged all the verities that had underpinned Canadian ideas about global politics and Canada's place in the world that had remained largely unchanged – and unchallenged – since the end of the Second World War in 1945.

Central to that vision was a global leadership role for the United States. As the Second World War came to an end, Canadian policy-makers, like their European counterparts, hoped that the United States would not retreat into the kind of isolationism that had marked the interwar years. Rather, they hoped that Americans would remain active in global politics, using the superordinate military and economic capabilities of the United States to maintain the security of Western Europe against the Soviet Union. The willingness of Americans to commit American military power to protect Europe and American economic capacity to rebuild Europe's shattered economies was seen in Ottawa as the foundation of Canada's security. Likewise, American leadership in shaping the post-war international order in a range of spheres was welcomed by Canadian policy-makers (even if they might have grumbled on occasion about how Americans chose to exercise that leadership).

A second verity that shaped Canadian approaches to global politics in the seventy-five years after 1945 held that in global politics Canada was always aligned geo-strategically with the United States. The U.S. was acknowledged as the leader of a series of interrelated military alliances ranged against the Soviet Union, and, after 1949, the People's Republic of China. Thus Canadians were stationed alongside American troops in Western Europe as part of the contribution to the North Atlantic Treaty Organization (NATO), a commitment that changed shape over the years but is still evident in how and where Canada deploys its armed forces. It was reflected in Canada's persistent attachment to the

'Five Eyes' (FVEY) intelligence alliance that binds Australia, Britain, Canada, New Zealand and the United States.

To be sure, Canadian alliance 'followership' was never absolute. Over the years governments in Ottawa, both Liberal and Conservative, found reasons to diverge from the alliance leader. Moreover, from the early 1960s on, some Canadians embraced the idea that their country should more properly be neutral in world politics, caught unhappily in the middle between the superpowers. But, while we have seen the slow evanescence of the idea of strategic partnership (Nossal, 2011), from the broader perspective of seven and a half decades, what is extraordinary is the degree to which Canada – and Canadians – remained committed to America's alliances and American leadership (Jockel & Sokolsky, 2009).

Canada's alignment went well beyond security, however. A third verity was the idea that multilateralism and multilateral organisations were a crucial part of the contemporary global order. For Canada, as for other small states in global politics, multilateralism remained the preferred approach for dealing with global issues. The creation and maintenance of multilateral institutions – as varied as the United Nations, the Commonwealth, la Francophonie, the G7, the G20 – that are able to develop, through global consensus, a rules-based approach to global governance has been seen by Canadians and other small countries for at least the last seventy-five years as a crucial mechanism for resolving the conflicts that will always be a feature of politics at a global level. Canadians have likewise always backed American leadership in the creation – and maintenance – of the range of multilateral organisations and arrangements that comprised the global order of both the Cold War and the post-Cold War eras (Keating, 2013).

Trump's election struck at all of these core foundations. For the first time since 1945, American voters had elected a president who unapologetically and unambiguously called into question both the liberal international order that the United States brought into being after 1945 and America's ongoing role in maintaining that order. Trump was openly dismissive of NATO, both in public and in private; he appeared to think of America's alliances as little more than grubby protection rackets, where smaller states are assumed to 'owe' huge sums of money to the United States directly for protection provided to them over the years. In addition, Trump's open denigration of the U.S. intelligence community and his politicisation of intelligence jeopardised the FVEY intelligence alliance (Lapointe, 2020).

Trump was also unremittingly critical of multilateralism as an approach to United States foreign policy, believing that foreigners have basically screwed Americans over the years by taking advantage of the United States via multilateral institutions and processes. His inaugural address (White House, 2017a) announcing his 'America First' policy reflected those long-held beliefs. As a corollary of his antipathy to multilateralism, Trump was particularly critical of international trade. A confirmed mercantilist and economic nationalist, Trump saw trade deficits as indications of national weakness, and his 'America First' policy was protectionist and driven by economic nationalism. As he famously tweeted, 'trade wars are good and easy to win' (Trump, 2018). Trade wars with America's trading partners, both threatened and actual, became a defining mark of his administration.

But Trump's critique of multilateralism was not just materialist. He had also always demonstrated a long-standing preoccupation with being laughed at that went back to the

1980s, when he had bought a newspaper ad calling for a new approach to international trade. 'The world is laughing at America's politicians,' the ad claimed. 'Let's not let our great country be laughed at anymore' (Trump, 1987). As president thirty years later, Trump persistently returned to this theme. In his telling, the United States had been 'demeaned' and treated unfairly; other countries and their leaders were always 'laughing at us,' as he put it in June 2017 (BBC News, 2017; Bump, 2017).

It was thus no surprise that as president, Trump moved to abandon as many multilateral engagements as he could. One of his first actions as president in January 2017 was to withdraw the United States from the Trans-Pacific Partnership, a free trade agreement that Washington itself had taken a lead in shaping. He withdrew from the Paris climate accord, claiming that the agreement was 'simply the latest example of Washington entering into an agreement that disadvantages the United States to the exclusive benefit of other countries' (White House, 2017b). His administration sought to undermine the World Trade Organization by refusing to fill vacant seats on the WTO's Appellate Body, a move that *Forbes* magazine characterised as an attempt to 'vandalise' the WTO (Brinkley, 2017). He seemed to take particular pleasure in disrupting two key summit meetings that always undergird the American-led multilateral order: the G7 and the NATO summits.

In short, in its first three years the Trump administration disrupted and destabilised global politics (Haas, 2020). Indeed, the speed with which America's role as the hegemon was undermined prompted Saideman (2017) to wonder whether that hoary staple of International Relations theory, hegemonic stability theory (for example, Webb & Krasner, 1989), should not be replaced by a new theory – 'hegemonic abdication theory.' However, as I have argued (Nossal, 2018), Trump was doing much more than just *abdicating* American global leadership; he was actively *ceding* leadership to others.

The COVID-19 pandemic accelerated all these trends. The Trump administration's chaotic response (Bowling et al., 2020) to the novel coronavirus pandemic – an admixture of denialism, obfuscation, ineptness and politicisation – was a key factor in shaping how the pandemic unfolded in the United States. The measures that were adopted by other communities – mask-wearing, social distancing and lockdowns of different varieties – were highly politicised in the United States by a president who refused to wear a mask, encouraged his followers to resist lockdowns, and continued to hold rallies marked by a lack of social distancing and mask-wearing until the very end of his presidency. It was thus no surprise that the United States, with some four percent of the world's population, should persistently have approximately 20% of the world's deaths from COVID-19, with an average of 951.8 deaths per day since the first reported death in February, and with weekly averages that spiked sharply upwards to over 1,400 deaths per day in November and December (COVID Tracking Project, 2020; Murphy et al., 2020).

The virulent spread of the disease across the United States had a major impact on American standing internationally. Many states banned American passport-holders altogether. Canada, which had originally negotiated a joint closing of the land border with the Trump administration for a thirty-day period in March, has extended the closure every month since then. Extending the closure yet again in October, Trudeau claimed that 'The U.S. is not in a place where we would feel comfortable reopening those borders,' and committed to keep the border closed until the United States had COVID-19 under control (Deerwester, 2020). Despite the loss of business from American tourists, public opinion in Canada strongly supported the prime minister's stand: one poll conducted in September revealed that fully 90% of Canadians agreed with keeping the border with the United States closed to non-essential travel (S. Harris, 2020).

The runaway spikes in infections and the high death rate produced another impact overseas. As Fintan O'Toole, a columnist for the *Irish Times*, wrote in a widely-circulated column in April 2020, 'the United States has stirred a very wide range of feelings in the rest of the world: love and hatred, fear and hope, envy and contempt, awe and anger. But there is one emotion that has never been directed towards the US until now: pity' (O'Toole, 2020). Fiona Hill, who had served as Trump's adviser on Russia, echoed that sentiment: she claimed in an interview with CNN that Americans 'are increasingly seen as an object of pity, including by our allies, because they are so shocked at what's happening internally, how we're eating ourselves alive with our divisions' (Yeo, 2020). That shock was nicely reflected in Trudeau's reaction when asked what he thought of Trump's approach to protestors. He paused for 21 long seconds, twice started to speak, and then stopped and groaned. Eventually he responded: 'We all watch in horror and consternation what's going on in the United States' (Tasker, 2020b).

The reaction of others in the international system at America's dysfunctional politics and chaotic administration had a mirror dynamic in the United States, however. The Trump administration actively avoided the kind of leadership that the United States had exercised in recent global crises, such as the Global Financial Crisis of 2008–2009, or the 2014 Ebola crisis, for example. Indeed, not only did the Trump administration refuse to take the lead in forging a multilateral response, but it engaged in a number of unilateral acts of abandonment. For example, it offered a German firm, Cure-Vac, USD1 billion to buy exclusive American monopoly rights to a COVID-19 vaccine (Hernández-Morales, 2020); it ordered an American firm, 3 M, to stop sending N95 masks to Canada (McCarten, 2020); and it refused to join a World Health Organization initiative on a vaccine (Rauhala & Abutaleb, 2020). More importantly, the Trump administration actively attacked the World Health Organization in a series of steps: in April, it suspended payments to the WHO; in May, it issued a series of threats to the WHO, demanding reforms, and threatening to leave; and in July, it gave notice of its intention to withdraw from the organisation in 2021 (Rauhala et al., 2020).

If Trump's retreat from multilateralism increasingly left Canada without its reliable anchors in global politics, Trump's other geostrategic moves also left Canada alone in the world. This was particularly true of relations with China. After Trump came to office in 2016, relations with the People's Republic of China grew increasingly fractious, partly because of Beijing's new assertiveness after Xi Jinping came to power in 2012–13; partly because of a growing consensus in official Washington that efforts to engage China in its rise to great power status were not working; but mostly because Trump's candidacy in 2015–16 had been in part built on bashing China for 'taking advantage' of Americans in the area of trade. As a result, in his first three years in office Trump himself devoted considerable efforts to 'making China pay' through the imposition of tariffs (that, of course, Americans, not the Chinese, paid for) and the negotiation of a trade agreement. In addition, the U.S. Department of Defense and the national security adviser ensured that the idea that China (and the Russian Federation) were 'revisionist' powers that were seeking a world antithetical to the interests of the United States was entrenched in the

2017 iteration of the National Security Strategy (United States, 2017, p. 25). The Trump administration also continued its long-standing dispute with Huawei Technologies, a Chinese information and communications technology company seeking to land a predominant place in the global market for the provision of 5G technology for broadband cellular networks. By 2019, the *Los Angeles Times* was characterising the moves against Huawei as a 'war' in which the U.S. was 'trying to destroy China's most successful brand' (Pearlstine et al., 2019).

Canada had already been affected by these efforts before the pandemic. On 1 December 2018, at the request of the United States, Canada arrested Meng Wanzhou, Huawei's chief financial officer and daughter of the firm's founder, Ren Zhengfei, as she was passing through Vancouver from Hong Kong to Mexico City. On 10 December, Chinese authorities arrested two Canadian citizens, Michael Kovrig and Michael Spavor, and have held them as hostages since then in retaliation for the Meng arrest. The very next day, Trump said in an interview that he would interfere in the Meng case 'if I think it's good for what will be certainly be the largest trade deal ever made' (Mason & Holland, 2018). While Trump may not have even been aware of the 'two Michaels' when he made his comments, his administration did virtually nothing to assist Canada in this case (Rauhala, 2019).

The COVID-19 pandemic accelerated tensions between Washington and Beijing, particularly after early reciprocal accusations about the origin of the coronavirus. Chinese officials claimed, without evidence, that U.S. service members visiting Wuhan for the Military World Games had brought COVID-19 with them (Myers, 2020); for his part, Trump claimed, equally without evidence, that the coronavirus originated in a lab in Wuhan (Singh et al., 2020). Trump then escalated his rhetorical attacks against China for the pandemic, calling COVID-19 the 'plague from China,' 'kung flu,' and 'Wuhan virus.' Indeed, Washington's insistence that the phrase 'Wuhan virus' be included in the joint statement of a summit of G7 foreign ministers prompted the summit to abandon a final communique (Simpson & Panetta, 2020). But the tension was more than rhetorical: over the course of 2020, Washington and Beijing engaged in tit-for-tat sanctions against each other (Ruwitch & Dahiya, 2020). For Canada, the radical escalation in Sino-American tensions during the pandemic highlighted the degree to which the evolving geostrategic environment leaves Canada vulnerable to the emerging great-power competition.

Conclusion

In 2019, Chrystia Freeland, then Canada's foreign minister, admitted to *The Economist* ('Canada in the global jungle,' 2019) that one of her favourite books was Robert Kagan's (2018) *The Jungle Grows Back*, which argued that the liberal world order 'is fragile and impermanent. Like a garden, it is ever under siege from the natural forces of history, the jungle whose vines and weeds constantly threaten to overwhelm it' (p. 4). By 2020, Trudeau had promoted Freeland to be deputy prime minister and minister of finance, but the jungle she was concerned about in 2019 continued to bedevil Canada. The COVID-19 pandemic accelerated a geostrategic shift that had started many years earlier. The election of Donald J. Trump in 2016 confirmed Zakaria's (2012) prediction that the 'post-American world' would soon arrive, even if Zakaria could not have anticipated that the post-American era he sketched would have been ushered in by the U.S. president himself.

Such developments have left Canada in a fraught place geopolitically. As Paris (2020) has noted, the world is less rule-bound and nastier, and those developments 'jeopardize Canadian interests in ways that may be unfamiliar to a country long used to a more benign international environment'. For Paris, and for many others besides (see the interviews in Ayed, 2019), the key for Canada in meeting the challenges of a post-pandemic world is to double down on multilateralism, to work not only with like-minded friends but to find, and work with, as many partners as possible. As Paris argued in a reflection on Canada's disputes with China and Saudi Arabia written before the pandemic, Canada has the ability to rally support, suggesting that 'it is not destined to be alone' (Paris, 2019).

To be sure, the victory of Joe Biden and the Democrats in November 2020 promises to slow, and perhaps even reverse, some of the geostrategic trends identified in this essay. It is likely that a Biden administration will deal more successfully with the COVID-19 pandemic. But even if the pandemic recedes in 2021–22 with the introduction of effective vaccines, it is doubtful that the multilateralism that is so widely seen as the buttress of Canada's geostrategic position in the 2020s will return. Four years of Trump's attacks on multilateralism and his abandonment of American leadership will likely have longer-term consequences. Even if the Biden administration seeks to turn the clock back and tries to resuscitate American leadership and nurture the 'garden' of multilateralism, it is likely that the attachment to Trumpism in the United States will linger long after Trump's departure. After all, over 74 million Americans – some 47% of U.S. voters – decided that they wanted four more years of Trumpism. We do not know precisely how many of those voters agreed with the Trumpian idea, so clearly articulated by two of his senior officials early in his presidency, that there is no such thing as a community of states in world politics (McMaster & Cohn, 2017), but we can conclude that this particular element of Trumpism will continue to run deep in American politics into the future.

Such a persistence of Trumpian ideas will likely continue to have an impact on American foreign policy. While the Biden administration may bring greater strategic coherence to great-power politics, it is likely that the relationship between the United States and China will continue its downward trend as a result of reciprocal and mirror dynamics in both countries. In the United States, Trump's defeat will not lessen the broad bipartisan support in Congress and widespread support among the American public for a hard line on China. In Beijing, the continuation of a hard line from the U.S. will merely confirm the view that the United States continues to be determined to frustrate China's rise, which in turn will prompt the leadership to double down on the 'wolf warrior' assertiveness and the appeals to Han nationalism that have been such a trademark of the leadership of Xi Jinping, particularly in the Indo-Pacific region. This will have major implications for all of the present friends and allies of the United States in the Indo-Pacific region, as they move to enhance their security in the face of the assertion of Chinese power.

And elsewhere in the international system, even those who might have yearned for a return to the era of American leadership during the Trump era will never be sure that Americans will not once again embrace a Trumpian alternative (Erlanger, 2020). It is likely that other states will increasingly find ways to 'take our destiny into our own hands,' as Angela Merkel, chancellor of Germany, put it just months after Trump's inauguration (Henley, 2017).

If this dynamic occurs across both the Atlantic and the Pacific, as America's allies in Europe and the Indo-Pacific regions move to cope with security challenges in their neighbourhoods created by the collapse of American leadership, that will, *pace* Paris, leave Canada very much alone in the world. Because Canada remains so firmly rooted – by its geography, its history, its economy, and its politics – in North America, Canadians are likely to find themselves in the same geostrategic location they were at the beginning of the twentieth century. This was a world in which multilateralism and global governance were so rudimentary and undeveloped that words to describe these activities had not even been thought of. Instead, world politics was dominated by great-power competition. In this world, Canada might have been alone with the United States in North America, but that solitary existence was leavened by Canada's membership in a hegemonic empire. In the twenty-first century, by contrast, with the likely evanescence of all those multilateral links beyond North America, Canadians will truly be left all alone with the United States.

Disclosure statement

No potential conflict of interest was reported by the author.

References

Authier, P. (2020, March 13). Quebec shuts down as premier François Legault declares an emergency. *Montreal Gazette*. https://montrealgazette.com/news/quebec/COVID-19-quebec-asks-anyone-returning-from-travel-to-self-quarantine/

Ayed, N. (2019, November 25). *Canada as a middle power in an upended world: Time for a foreign policy reset?* CBC Radio: Ideas. https://www.cbc.ca/radio/ideas/canada-as-a-middle-power-in-an-upended-world-time-for-a-foreign-policy-reset-1.5372192

BBC News. (2017, June 2). Trump: World won't laugh any more. *BBC News*. https://www.bbc.com/news/av/world-us-canada-40128556

Berthiaume, L. (2020, September 22). Majority of Canadians support wearing masks during COVID-19, poll suggests. *Toronto Star*. https://www.thestar.com/news/canada/2020/09/22/majority-of-canadians-support-wearing-masks-during-COVID-19-poll-suggests.html

Boucher, J.-C. (2020, June 17). Canada's failed Security Council bid marks the death of our traditional foreign policy. *National Post*. https://nationalpost.com/opinion/jean-christophe-boucher-canadas-failed-security-council-bid-marks-the-death-of-our-traditional-foreign-policy

Bowling, C. J., Fisk, J. M., & Morris, C. J. (2020). Seeking patterns in chaos: Transactional federalism in the Trump administration's response to the COVID-19 pandemic. *American Review of Public Administration*, *50*(6–7), 512–518. https://doi.org/10.1177/0275074020941686

Brinkley, J. (2017, November 27). *Trump is quietly trying to vandalize the WTO*. Forbes. https://www.forbes.com/sites/johnbrinkley/2017/11/27/trump-quietly-trying-to-vandalize-the-wto/

Bump, P. (2017, June 28). Trump's pledge to keep the world from laughing at us hits another setback. *Washington Post*. https://www.washingtonpost.com/news/politics/wp/2017/06/28/trumps-pledge-to-keep-the-world-from-laughing-at-us-hits-another-setback/

Burney, D. H., & Hampson, F. O. (2020). *Braver Canada: Shaping our destiny in a precarious world*. McGill-Queen's University Press.

Canada. (2020). *Coronavirus disease (COVID-19): Outbreak update [Updated daily]*. Government of Canada. https://www.canada.ca/en/public-health/services/diseases/2019-novel-coronavirus-infection.html

Canada in the global jungle: A mid-sized democracy copes with a forbidding new environment. (2019, February 9). *The Economist*. https://www.economist.com/the-americas/2019/02/09/canada-in-the-global-jungle

Canadian Border Services Agency. (2020, March 17). *Border tips for returning Canadian snowbirds [News release]*. https://www.canada.ca/en/border-services-agency/news/2020/03/border-tips-for-returning-canadian-snowbirds.html

Cecco, L. (2020a, March 13). Justin Trudeau announces sweeping steps to tackle coronavirus in Canada. *The Guardian*. https://www.theguardian.com/world/2020/mar/13/justin-trudeau-coronavirus-response-canada-measures

Cecco, L. (2020b, March 16). 'Stay home': Justin Trudeau closes Canada's borders over coronavirus. *The Guardian*. https://www.theguardian.com/world/2020/mar/16/justin-trudeau-closes-canada-borders-coronavirus

COVID Tracking Project. (2020). *US daily deaths [Data updated daily]*. https://COVIDtracking.com/data/charts/us-daily-deaths

Davidson, S. (2020, March 17). Ontario declares state of emergency amid COVID-19 pandemic. *CTV News*. https://toronto.ctvnews.ca/ontario-declares-state-of-emergency-amid-COVID-19-pandemic-1.4856033

Deerwester, J. (2020, October 15). Justin Trudeau: Canada-US border will stay closed until America gets COVID-19 under control. *USA Today*. https://www.usatoday.com/story/travel/news/2020/10/15/justin-trudeau-canada-us-border-not-reopening-COVID-19/3661758001/

Drezner, D. W. (2020, May 11). So what do international relations scholars think about COVID-19 and world politics? *Washington Post*. https://www.washingtonpost.com/outlook/2020/05/11/so-what-do-international-relations-scholars-think-about-COVID-19-world-politics/

Elliott, J. K. (2020, April 8). Trudeau cringes at his own 'speaking moistly' tip for coronavirus masks. *Global News*. https://globalnews.ca/news/6792967/coronavirus-trudeau-speaking-moistly/

Erlanger, S. (2020, October 22). Europe wonders if it can rely on U.S. again, whoever wins. *New York Times*. https://www.nytimes.com/2020/10/22/world/europe/europe-biden-trump-diplomacy.html

Grant, K. (2020, June 25). 81% of COVID-19 deaths in Canada were in long-term care—nearly double OECD average. *Globe and Mail*. https://www.theglobeandmail.com/canada/article-new-data-show-canada-ranks-among-worlds-worst-for-ltc-deaths/

Greenhill, R., & Welsh, J. M. (2020a, September 1). *Reframing Canada's global engagement: Ten strategic choices for decision-makers*. Global Canada. https://global-canada.org/wp-content/uploads/2020/09/Ten-Strategic-Choices-August-2020-2.pdf

Greenhill, R., & Welsh, J. M. (2020b, September 1). *Reframing Canada's global engagement: A diagnostic of key trends and sources of influence*. Global Canada. https://global-canada.org/wp-content/uploads/2020/09/A-Diagnostic-of-Key-Trends-August-2020.pdf

Haas, R. (2020). Present at the disruption: How Trump unmade US foreign policy. *Foreign Affairs*, *99*(5), 24–34. https://www.foreignaffairs.com/articles/united-states/2020-08-11/present-disruption

Harris, K. (2020, March 5). Trudeau says 'knee-jerk reactions' won't stop spread of COVID-19. *CBC News*. https://www.cbc.ca/news/politics/COVID19-trudeau-coronavirus-travel-1.5486799

Harris, S. (2020, September 15). Why many Canadians support the Canada-U.S. border closure, despite the costs. *CBC News*. https://www.cbc.ca/news/business/canada-u-s-border-closure-support-mayors-tourism-trump-1.5722974

Henley, J. (2017, May 28). Angela Merkel: EU cannot completely rely on US and Britain any more. *The Guardian*. https://www.theguardian.com/world/2017/may/28/merkel-says-eu-cannot-completely-rely-on-us-and-britain-any-more-g7-talks

Hernández-Morales, A. (2020, March 15). Germany confirms that Trump tried to buy firm working on coronavirus vaccine. *Politico*. https://www.politico.eu/article/germany-confirms-that-donald-trump-tried-to-buy-firm-working-on-coronavirus-vaccine/

Ibbitson, J. (2020, April 11). Emergency wage subsidy approved, but parties dispute how parliament should meet next. *Globe and Mail*. https://www.theglobeandmail.com/politics/article-house-approves-emergency-wage-subsidy-dispute-how-to-meet-in-future/

Jackson, E. B., Parajon, E., Peterson, S., Powers, R., & Tierney, M. J. (2020). *TRIP snap poll XIII*. Teaching, Research & International Policy (TRIP) Project. https://trip.wm.edu/data/our-surveys/snap-polls/Snap_Poll_13_Report_Final.pdf

Jockel, J. T., & Sokolsky, J. J. (2009). Canada and NATO: Keeping Ottawa in, expenses down, criticism out ... and the country secure. *International Journal*, *64*(2), 315–336. https://doi.org/10.1177/002070200906400202

Jones, A. M. (2020, March 23). More than a million Canadians and permanent residents return from abroad amid COVID-19 warnings. *CTV News*. https://www.ctvnews.ca/health/coronavirus/more-than-a-million-canadians-and-permanent-residents-return-from-abroad-amid-COVID-19-warnings-1.4865042

Juneau, T. (2020, June 7). Canada will pay the price for neglecting our foreign policy. *Globe and Mail*. https://www.theglobeandmail.com/opinion/article-canada-will-pay-the-price-for-neglecting-our-foreign-policy/

Kagan, R. (2018). *The jungle grows back: America and our imperiled world*. Alfred A. Knopf.

Keating, T. (2013). *Canada and world order: The multilateralist tradition in Canadian foreign policy* (3rd ed.). Oxford University Press.

Lapointe, M. (2020, September 14). Experts sound alarm over 'politicized' U.S. intelligence, say COVID-19 pandemic a 'wake-up call' about Canada's new national security threats. *Hill Times*. https://www.hilltimes.com/2020/09/14/experts-sound-alarm-over-politicized-u-s-intelligence-say-covid-19-pandemic-a-wake-up-call-about-new-national-security-threats/263278

Mason, J., & Holland, S. (2018, December 11). *Exclusive: Trump says he would intervene in U.S. case against Huawei CFO*. Reuters. https://www.reuters.com/article/us-usa-trump-huawei-tech-exclusive-idUSKBN1OA2PQ

McCarten, J. (2020, April 3). 3M says Trump officials have told it to stop sending face masks to Canada. Trudeau responds. *National Post*. https://nationalpost.com/news/world/3m-says-trump-officials-have-told-it-to-stop-sending-face-masks-to-canada

McMaster, H. R., & Cohn, G. D. (2017, May 30). America First doesn't mean America alone. *Wall Street Journal*. https://www.wsj.com/articles/america-first-doesnt-mean-america-alone-1496187426

Murphy, J., Wu, J., Chiwaya, N., & Muccari, R. (2020) Coronavirus deaths in the U.S., per day [Graphic updated daily]. *NBC News*. https://www.nbcnews.com/health/health-news/coronavirus-deaths-united-states-each-day-2020-n1177936

Mustapha, J., & Van Rythoven, E. (2020, July 31). *Love, loathing, and loss: America's COVID-19 response and the view from Canada*. Duck of Minerva. https://duckofminerva.com/2020/07/love-loathing-and-loss-americas-COVID-19-response-and-the-view-from-canada.html

Myers, S. L. (2020, March 13). China spins tale that the U.S. Army started the coronavirus epidemic. *New York Times*. https://www.nytimes.com/2020/03/13/world/asia/coronavirus-china-conspiracy-theory.html

Nossal, K. R. (2011). America's 'most reliable ally'? Canada and the evanescence of the culture of partnership. In G. Anderson & C. Sands (Eds.), *Forgotten partnership redux: Canada-U.S. relations in the 21st century* (pp. 375–404). Cambria Press.

Nossal, K. R. (2018, November 12). *The Trump cession and the dismantling of American hegemony*. https://nossalk.org/2018/11/12/the-trump-cession/

Nye, J. S., Jr. (2020, April 16). No, the coronavirus will not change the global order. *Foreign Policy*. https://foreignpolicy.com/2020/04/16/coronavirus-pandemic-china-united-states-power-competition/

O'Toole, F. (2020, April 25). Donald Trump has destroyed the country he promised to make great again. *Irish Times*. https://www.irishtimes.com/opinion/fintan-o-toole-donald-trump-has-destroyed-the-country-he-promised-to-make-great-again-1.4235928

Paris, R. (2019). Alone in the world? Making sense of Canada's disputes with Saudi Arabia and China. *International Journal*, *74*(1), 151–161. https://doi.org/10.1177/0020702019834652

Paris, R. (2020, July 16). *Navigating the new world disorder: Canada's post-pandemic foreign policy*. Public Policy Forum. https://ppforum.ca/publications/navigating-the-new-world-disorder/

Pearlstine, N., Krishnakumar, P., & Pierson, D. (2019, December 19). The war against Huawei: Why the U.S. is trying to destroy China's most successful brand. *Los Angeles Times*. https://www.latimes.com/projects/la-fg-huawei-timeline/

Public Health Agency of Canada. (2020). *From risk to resilience: An equity approach to COVID-19 —The chief public health officer of Canada's report on the state of public health in Canada 2020*. https://www.canada.ca/content/dam/phac-aspc/documents/corporate/publications/chief-public-health-officer-reports-state-public-health-canada/from-risk-resilience-equity-approach-covid-19/cpho-covid-report-eng.pdf

Rabson, M. (2020, June 5). Ottawa offers $14-billion to provincial and territorial governments for COVID-19 relief efforts. *Globe and Mail*. https://www.theglobeandmail.com/politics/article-trudeau-to-offer-premiers-billions-to-help-reopen-provincial-and/

Rauch, J. (2016, July/August). How American politics went insane. *The Atlantic*. https://www.theatlantic.com/magazine/archive/2016/07/how-american-politics-went-insane/485570/

Rauhala, E. (2019, May 8). Canada arrested Huawei's Meng for the United States. As China retaliates, it's on its own. *Washington Post*. https://www.washingtonpost.com/world/the_americas/canada-helped-the-us-arrest-meng-wanzhou-as-it-gets-punished-by-china-its-on-its-own/2019/05/07/c8152fbe-6d18-11e9-bbe7-1c798fb80536_story.html

Rauhala, E., & Abutaleb, Y. (2020, September 1). U.S. says it won't join WHO-linked effort to develop, distribute coronavirus vaccine. *Washington Post*. https://www.washingtonpost.com/world/coronavirus-vaccine-trump/2020/09/01/b44b42be-e965-11ea-bf44-0d31c85838a5_story.html

Rauhala, E., Demirjian, K., & Olorunnipa, T. (2020, July 7). Trump administration sends letter withdrawing U.S. from World Health Organization over coronavirus response. *Washington Post*. https://www.washingtonpost.com/world/trump-united-states-withdrawal-world-health-organization-coronavirus/2020/07/07/ae0a25e4-b550-11ea-9a1d-d3db1cbe07ce_story.html

Ruwitch, J., & Dahiya, N. (2020, July 22). *Timeline: The unraveling of U.S.-China relations*. NPR. https://www.npr.org/2020/07/22/893767828/timeline-the-unraveling-of-u-s-china-relations

Saideman, S. M. (2017, December 10). *Hegemonic abdication theory*. Saideman's semi-spew. http://saideman.blogspot.com/2017/12/hegemonic-abdication-theory.html

Simpson, K., & Panetta, A. (2020, March 25). G7 ministers spike joint statement on COVID-19 after U.S. demands it be called 'Wuhan virus.' *CBC News*. https://www.cbc.ca/news/politics/g7-COVID-19-coronavirus-wuhan-pompeo-trump-1.5510329

Singh, M., Davison, H., & Borger, J. (2020, May 1). Trump claims to have evidence coronavirus started in Chinese lab but offers no details. *The Guardian*. https://www.theguardian.com/us-news/2020/apr/30/donald-trump-coronavirus-chinese-lab-claim

Tam, T. [@CPHO_Canada]. (2020, January 26). *3/3 there is no clear evidence that this virus is spread easily from person to person. The risk to Canadians remains low*. Twitter. https://twitter.com/CPHO_Canada/status/1221606834987053056

Tasker, J. P. (2020a, March 17). Canadian snowbirds told to come home as some insurers warn medical insurance will be restricted. *CBC News*. https://www.cbc.ca/news/politics/canadian-snowbirds-COVID-19-insurance-1.5499666

Tasker, J. P. (2020b, June 2). *Trudeau says Canadians watching U.S. events in 'horror,' avoids naming Trump after long pause*. CBC News. https://www.cbc.ca/news/politics/trudeau-trump-george-floyd-1.5594918; https://www.youtube.com/watch?v=SeaDi-0Nz8w

Trudeau, J. (2020, March 18). *Prime Minister's remarks announcing the COVID-19 economic response plan*. Justin Trudeau, Prime Minister of Canada. https://pm.gc.ca/en/news/speeches/2020/03/18/prime-ministers-remarks-announcing-COVID-19-economic-response-plan

Trump, D. [@realDonaldTrump]. (2018, March 2). *When a country (USA) is losing many billions of dollars on trade with virtually every country it does business with, trade wars are good and easy to win.* Twitter. https://twitter.com/realDonaldTrump/status/969525362580484098

Trump, D. J. (1987, September 2). There's nothing wrong America's foreign defense policy that a little backbone can't cure [Advertisement]. *New York Times*, p. A28. https://timesmachine.nytimes.com/timesmachine/1987/09/02/issue.html

United States. (2017). *National security strategy of the United States of America.* President of the U.S. https://www.whitehouse.gov/wp-content/uploads/2017/12/NSS-Final-12-18-2017-0905-2.pdf

Van der Linden, C. (2020, August 12). *Canada is not immune to the politics of coronavirus masks.* The Conversation. https://theconversation.com/canada-is-not-immune-to-the-politics-of-coronavirus-masks-144110

Webb, M. C., & Krasner, S. D. (1989). Hegemonic stability theory: An empirical assessment. *Review of International Studies, 15*(2), 183–198. https://doi.org/10.1017/S0260210500112999

White House. (2017a, January 20). *Inaugural address.* https://www.whitehouse.gov/briefings-statements/the-inaugural-address/

White House. (2017b, June 1). *Statement by President Trump on the Paris climate accord.* Ditto. https://www.whitehouse.gov/briefings-statements/statement-president-trump-paris-climate-accord/

World Health Organization (WHO). (2020, March 11). *Coronavirus disease 2019 (COVID-19) situation report – 51.* https://www.who.int/docs/default-source/coronaviruse/situation-reports/20200311-sitrep-51-COVID-19.pdf

Woods, M. (2020, May 20). Canada's new coronavirus face mask rules: What you need to know. *Huffington Post.* https://www.huffingtonpost.ca/entry/canada-mask-rules-theresa-tam_ca_5ec5b0c0c5b62653f79ff80f

Worldometer. (2020). *COVID-19 coronavirus pandemic [Updated daily].* https://www.worldometers.info/coronavirus/

Yeo, P. K. (2020, September 22). *Trump's former Russia adviser: U.S. increasingly seen as 'object of pity.'* Daily Beast. https://www.thedailybeast.com/former-trump-russia-adviser-fiona-hill-us-increasingly-seen-as-object-of-pity

Zakaria, F. (2012). *The post-American world: Release 2.0.* W.W. Norton & Company.

India's domestic and foreign policy responses to COVID-19

Pradeep Taneja and Azad Singh Bali

ABSTRACT

A year after the first known case of COVID-19 was reported, India had the second-highest incidence of cases and accounted for about 13% of the global total. This article traces India's local and foreign policy responses to the global pandemic. The article advances two arguments. First, while the government was swift and decisive in its response, the pandemic exposed weakness in policy coordination and inadequacies in India's social protection system. Second, while the pandemic spread rapidly across the country, the government exploited diplomatic opportunities to demonstrate leadership both within South Asia and globally.

Introduction

Like most other countries, India was ill-prepared to deal with the outbreak of SARS-COV-2 or the COVID-19 pandemic. Its health care system has been overburdened and the societal fault lines have been brought into sharper relief by the virus. Its relatively early response to the pandemic, including a national lockdown, might have delayed the full-scale impact of the pandemic but it could not escape the ravages of the disease on its social, economic and political life. A year after the first reported case of the virus, India had about 10 million cases accounting for 13% of the global total. This headline number, however, masks the relatively low number of cases once adjusted for population; a relatively low case fatality rate of 1.45 (i.e. number of deaths per 100 infections); and a relatively high recovery rate of 95%. This paper does not speak to India's performance on these benchmark indicators. Instead, the focus is to document India's policy responses to the pandemic. The paper is divided into two main parts. The first part examines the domestic responses to the pandemic, including the lockdown and the resultant migrant worker crisis, economic interventions and the health policy response. In the second part, the foreign policy initiatives taken by the Indian government to deal with the challenging international environment in the wake of the pandemic are examined.

Domestic response

India recorded its first case of coronavirus on 30 January 2020 when a student who had just returned from the epicentre of the global pandemic in Wuhan tested positive for the virus. In the following days India introduced a number of precautionary measures including thermal checks at ports of entry and requiring overseas arrivals to share their travel histories. As cases continued to gradually increase over the ensuing weeks in February, the government banned international arrivals from countries with high rates of infection including China, Turkey, the European Union, Malaysia and Afghanistan among others (Ganpathy, 2020a). This was followed by a ban on all international flights to India for a week starting in the middle of March (Ganpathy, 2020b).

Nationwide lockdown

The series of gradual restrictions imposed through February and March culminated on 24 March in the first of what would be a series of nationwide lockdowns (Gettleman & Schultz, 2020). The decision to impose a lockdown was significant for several reasons. First, India was one of the first countries in the world to impose such a stark national response to the global pandemic. Second, in March India had a relatively small number of cases (about 500 odd infections compared to the global total of 450,000) (Coronavirus Resource Centre, 2020). Third, the lockdown was imposed with limited consultation or forewarning to citizens, industry or even government agencies. The lockdown was announced by Prime Minister Narendra Modi in an address to the nation on 23 March at 8 pm, and it was to come into effect at midnight. The Prime Minister's address focussed on the rationale for the lockdown, explaining its significance but offered little insight into the logistics or how it would be managed across 28 States and 8 Union Territories. Following the address, the Ministry of Home Affairs released guidelines on the lockdown and announced that essential services such as banking, finance and telecom would continue to function, and supermarkets, grocery stores and fruit and vegetable shops and chemists would remain open (Government of India, 2020). For its part, the government argued that its domestic policy response to the pandemic was influenced by a 'barbell' strategy. The aim of such an approach is to manage extreme uncertainty by hedging against adverse outcomes. Such an approach, it was argued, was necessary to manage the extreme uncertainty associated with the pandemic, and allow the government a knowledge base to design policy interventions as well as create capacity (Sanyal, 2020).

A key element of the government's response to the pandemic focussed on building a sense of solidarity and community among people. Prime Minister Modi used the aphorism, *Jaan Hai Toh Jahan Hai* (only if you live, you have the world ahead of you), aimed at uniting the people and engendering a sense of resolve to bring the spread of viral infection under control. In televised national addresses, the Prime Minister pleaded with businesses not to make their staff redundant, look out for vulnerable members of the community, and for individuals and companies to contribute to a newly established fund – The Prime Minister's Citizen Assistance and Relief in Emergency Situations Fund (shortened to PM-CARES Fund). The announcement of PM-CARES Fund was followed by a shallow and partisan debate in Parliament on the need, legal status, and transparency of the charitable fund (Business Today, 2020; The Wire, 2020; Venkat, 2020). In repeated addresses, the Prime Minister used his personal appeal to reiterate the importance of social distancing and wearing masks while in public. His messages, buttressed by a groundswell of public trust and political legitimacy, resonated with people in the initial stages of the lockdown.

While many heralded the government's decision as astute and bold, there was a sobering refrain of caution on the economic and social costs of a nationwide lockdown imposed with only four hours' notice. The lockdown was introduced without giving state governments and their district administrators time to prepare. This contributed to creating an environment of chaos and panic in the early days of the lockdown. A former member of the Prime Minister's Economic Advisory Council acknowledged that the nation-wide lockdown 'was a drastic measure for a country of 1.3 billion people ... but a pre-emptive necessary step' to build capacity (Ravi, 2020). Moreover, implementing such a decision in an expansive federal system – where responsibilities for key public services during a pandemic were distributed across central and state governments – is a challenging task (Debroy, 2020; Nageswaran, 2020b). Nonetheless, the government did not anticipate key developments in the aftermath of the lockdown, for example, the mass movement of migrant labour – discussed later in this section – or consult with state governments who are primarily responsible on issues related to migrant labour. For critics, the government's handling of the lockdown in many respects is characteristic of an emerging policy style where important implementation aspects of key policy decisions and flagship initiatives, such as the recent tax reforms (the Goods and Services Tax – GST) and the 2016 Demonetisation, are not adequately considered (Bardhan, 2020; Comptroller and Auditor General of India, 2019).

Domestic migrant labour crisis

There was widespread support across political parties for the nationwide lockdown and the swift action of the government. Despite this political support, the immediate impact of the nationwide lockdown was felt by millions of India's daily wage earners and those employed in the informal sector. As most businesses that employed millions of people were forced to close, migrant workers had to contend with the loss of income and uncertainty about their employment. With no income and no money to pay rent, large numbers of migrant workers began gathering at train and bus terminals looking to return to their native homes (Ranjan, 2020). The following weeks saw millions of migrant workers and their families making their way back home under abject conditions. Tens of thousands walked for hundreds of kilometres while others rode their bicycles on national highways in a rush to get home, as train and bus services were halted. The plight of the migrant families threw entrenched fault lines in India's social protection system into sharper relief. Despite recent efforts to improve social protection (Asher et al., 2015; Ramesh & Bali, 2021), those employed in the informal sector were particularly affected by the absence of a robust public health system, and inadequate labour market protections. It was only in the month of May that central and state governments rolled out special buses and trains to ferry migrant workers back to their villages and hometowns. For example, between May and June 15, about 4450 special trains were organised and used by six million migrant workers (*The Hindu*, 2020b). Most of these trains terminated in the populous states of Uttar Pradesh, Bihar, Jharkhand, and Madhya Pradesh and Odisha (*The Economic Times*, 2020b)

The migrant labour challenge was accentuated by the absence of reliable data on the number of migrant workers or their distribution across Indian states. The Economic Survey of India (2017, p. 267) estimates that the total size of the migrant workforce was about 100 million in 2016; and that inter-state migration between 2011–16 was approximately 9 million annually (The World Economic Forum, 2017). Debroy (2020) cites the Inter-State Migrant Workmen Act of 1979, which requires state governments to maintain data on migrants and key variables around their employment. However, successive state governments have failed to maintain comprehensive data on migrant workers (*Financial Express*, 2020). In similar vein, many state governments failed to maintain up to date databases on key variables that inform policy deliberations during a pandemic. For example, in 2018 the state of Bihar registered only about a third, and the state of Jharkand only about half of total deaths (Debroy, 2020). It is not unreasonable to expect that the lack of data constrained both policy deliberations around the decision to impose the lockdown and the measures adopted to mitigate the impact of the pandemic. For its part, the government has since announced its decision to create a nationwide database on migrant workers (*Financial Express*, 2020).

Social policy responses

The Finance Minister announced a COVID relief package of about INR 1.7 trillion or about US$22 billion on 26 March 2020. Most of this funding was focussed on food relief for identified families, as well as cash transfers to the elderly and a select group of families. This included, front loading income support to about 90 million farmers; raising wages under India's flagship rural employment guarantee programme (MGNREGA); a one-time payment of INR 1,000 to the elderly poor; a monthly payment of INR 500 for three months to about 200 million women; free cooking gas cylinders for 3 months to 80 million households; increasing the food allowance by 5 kilograms of wheat or rice for about 800 million individuals; and a host of regulatory interventions such as increasing the withdrawal limits in provident funds (Mishra, 2020). While the COVID relief package was well-received, analysts were quick to point out that most of the measures announced were commitments made by the government earlier. Indeed, Bajoria (2020) finds that the monetary value of additional commitments in the government's relief package was about INR 620 billion – far short of the amount claimed by the government.

A key element of the government's social policy response, in many respects echoing efforts made over the past five years (see Asher et al. (2015) for example), rests on reducing the administrative burdens in accessing social services. For example, the government announced the national portability of food entitlements it provides through the Public Distribution System (PDS) to identified households.

Continuation of lockdown

By the end of the first lockdown (March 24-April 14), there were about two million cases globally and India accounted for about 12,000 of them. The government extended the lockdown by three more weeks (April 15-May 3) with more discretion given to local authorities to manage restrictions in districts provided they were not considered infection 'hot spots'. By the end of April, the Ministry of Home Affairs allowed inter-state movement.

As local officials were given greater discretion in handling the restrictions within their administrative catchment areas, it allowed for different 'models' of pandemic response across India to appear. In the initial stages of the pandemic, Kerala's model which relied on extensive surveillance, tracking and tracing, containment and engaging with the community was heralded by the central government as a model for other state administrations to follow.

Similarly, local administrators in cities (for example, in Chandigarh) were entrepreneurial in offering their residents continued public services such as mobile ATMs throughout this period. However, these ideal-typical models in responding to the virus did not last long as the pandemic took hold and infections began to spread rapidly. There were about 42,000 cases in India by the end of the second lockdown, which prompted the government to extend it by two more weeks from May 4 to 17, and again from May 18 to May 31. During these time periods, the Indian government had largely devolved decision-making to state and local administrations. By May 31, the total number of cases in India had increased to about 190,000. The total number of cases continued to rise in the months of June through mid-September at an alarming rate, reaching 5.2 million at its peak.

Between the intervening months India's cumulative case total had increased 27-fold. Since then, the pandemic has grown rapidly and, by the middle of November 2020, there were 53.9 million cases worldwide and 1.31 million deaths. India was the second worst affected country after the United States, with more than 8.81 million cases and 129,635 deaths. These aggregate numbers however mask India's performance on other important indicators such as the case fatality rate and cases per million population. For example, data from the Ministry of Health and Family Welfare suggests that the case fatality rate as of mid-November was 1.5% significantly lower than other countries at similar levels of economic development. Similarly, India's cases per million population are among the lowest in the world (*The Hindu*, 2020c).

Economic interventions

The economic costs of bringing an already slowing economy to a grinding halt for 11 weeks continued to accumulate, and the government had little option but to lift restrictions and reopen the economy. In a series of gradual steps between June and October, the central and state governments removed restrictions, allowing economic activity to recommence. To mitigate the economic impact of the pandemic, the central government announced a series of reform measures under the slogan '*Atmanirbhar Bharat*' or self-reliant India. These reforms were announced in three tranches. Most of these were focussed on medium to long-term initiatives aimed at formalising labour markets, extending credit to farmers and industries, strengthening local markets, supply chains, and boosting domestic production. The reforms were layered with a series of actions aimed at lowering regulatory costs and administrative burdens, improving the ease of doing business, and attracting investment (Nageswaran, 2020a).

The monetary value of the economic reforms announced was about INR 20 trillion or US$260 billion (10% of India's GDP). It is too early to assess the efficacy of these reforms given the lags in economic interventions and ensuing economic activity. With negative growth in the first two quarters of the current fiscal year and diminished prospects for robust growth through the rest of the year, the Reserve Bank of India expects India's GDP to contract by 9.5% in the 2020–21 financial year (Saha, 2020). The Indian government has realised that it has limited options to boost economic growth but to revitalise economic activity by removing restrictions. India's economic responses to the pandemic (unlike those in the United States, Singapore and Australia, for example) were not aimed at boosting individual and household demand or protecting jobs by subsidising wages but instead focused on providing short term relief to poor households and introducing quasi-structural reforms that aim to crowd-in investment and economic growth in the medium-term. This is consistent with the government's overall approach to economic policymaking (Nageswaran, 2020a, 2020b).

Following the announcement made by the Finance Minister, India's central bank, the Reserve Bank of India, also announced a slew of monetary policy measures to increase liquidity in the markets.

Health policy responses

The Indian government has maintained that successive lockdowns allowed its health system sufficient time to gear up and boost capacity. India's health system, particularly its public health system, is fragmented and fractured. There are large variations in the capacity and quality of public hospitals and health centres across India (Bali & Ramesh, 2015). Starved of funds, these hospitals are often out of essential supplies and have been unable to recruit and retain adequate medical personnel. This collectively results in public hospitals generally providing relatively poor quality of care and largely servicing those who cannot afford private hospitals. Efforts to address these challenges began in earnest in 2018 with the launch of the Pradhan Mantri Jan Arogya Yojana (PM-JAY). PM-JAY is a public health insurance scheme that covers about 100 million poor families at empanelled public and private hospitals. The programme, however, does not cover India's growing middle class, is still in its infancy and therefore has done little to address the limited capacity of public hospitals.

The limited capacity of public hospitals to provide adequate care was a major constraint in India's ability to effectively respond to the pandemic. Private hospitals which provide an overwhelming share of ambulatory care in India were also overwhelmed in the initial stages of the pandemic. There were multiple reports of sick patients being denied treatment and being forced to visit multiple hospitals before receiving care. As private hospitals are poorly regulated, some hospitals responded by significantly increasing prices, as well as refusing to admit COVID-19 patients.

The government responded to these health policy challenges. First, it increased the capacity of public hospitals and health centres through increased funding to buy ventilators and therapeutics. Elective surgeries were delayed, and certain public hospitals were designated as COVID hospitals in catchment areas. Second, the government introduced price controls to curb opportunism by private hospitals. The Chief Minister of Delhi, for example, required private hospitals to publicly display their hospital bed capacity at the entrance of hospitals. Third, many state governments, for example, Maharashtra, 'took over' up to 80% of hospital beds in private hospitals (Sequeira, 2020).

The Indian government also launched *Aarogya Setu*, a contact tracing smartphone app that uses Bluetooth technology and location data to detect if a person has been in contact with a COVID-19 infected patient. In addition, a number of state governments have also launched apps with live information about the availability of hospital beds and ventilators in COVID-19 designated hospitals. There were, however, reports of inconsistencies between the data shown on the app and the actual availability of hospital beds, creating confusion and frustration among patients and their families (*The Hindu*, 2020a). Not only is the efficacy of these apps open to question, there have also been privacy concerns expressed by civil liberties groups (Centre for Internet and Society, 2020).

Another important health policy issue relates to India's capacity to produce vaccines, as well as administer the vaccine across its 1.3 billion citizens. India produces as much as 60% of the world's vaccines (The BBC, 2020), and many low- and middle-income countries rely on its production capacity. For example, the Serum Institute of India – the world's largest vaccine manufacturer – has entered into commercial agreements to produce over a billion doses of the vaccine developed by AstraZeneca and the University of Oxford once it receives regulatory approval (*Nature*, 2020). Agreements made with the Government of India require half of these vaccines to be earmarked to immunise vulnerable cohorts of the population in India, and in other low-income countries. Despite India's strong track record in the pharmaceutical sector, and its capacity to produce vaccines, there are many challenges in rolling out the vaccine across India. These challenges echo some of the health system constraints described earlier in the paper as well as issues around logistics, supply chain and maintaining cold chains (*The Washington Post*, 2020)

Recent research in the policy sciences has focused on the importance of policy capacity, learning, and the role of anticipation in developing effective policy responses (Bali et al., 2019; Capano et al., 2020). That is, the ability of governments to prepare, reflect on and draw lessons from past experiences, work across government agencies, and anticipate blind spots and vulnerabilities of certain population segments is critical to effective policymaking. By this yardstick, the Indian government's domestic response to the COVID-19 crisis has been a case of hit-and-miss. While the initial response was swift and decisive, it failed to take into account the consequences and side-effects of the actions taken. The most glaring failure of the government's response relates to the decision to impose a lockdown with only four hours' notice. It failed to anticipate and prepare for the adverse consequences of the lockdown on some of the most vulnerable people in society, especially domestic migrant workers. The Prime Minister initially took the lead in coordinating the response with the state governments and organising video conferences with the state Chief Ministers, but as the pandemic began to spread rapidly and the number of infections increased sharply, the Prime Minister seemed to shift the bulk of the responsibility for responding to the pandemic to the state governments. The absence of instruments to coordinate between government agencies, especially across central and state governments, in the areas of health and social policy, constrained India's efforts domestically to control the pandemic.

Similarly, Prime Minister Modi was centre stage in communicating directly with the people by addressing the nation seven times between 19 March and 20 October, but the length of his speeches grew shorter as the pandemic worsened; the last two speeches on 30 June and 20 October were far apart and lasted just 16 minutes and 13 minutes respectively, compared to some of his earlier speeches that ranged between 28 and 34 minutes (DNA, 2020). It is easy to understand why the prime minister took the lead in communicating directly with the people via television, radio and his social media accounts. The reason is his personal popularity, and it is likely that the people would pay more heed to the message if it was coming directly from the Prime Minister. While Mr Modi enjoys a groundswell of public trust and political capacity, much of his communication about the government's response to COVID-19 has, however, been in the form of monologues; unlike his counterparts in other democracies, Prime Minister Modi does not address press conferences and rarely agrees to media interviews.

The pandemic has raised several governance questions, particularly around lax enforcement of important statutes, the division of responsibilities across central and state governments during a pandemic, and instruments of policy coordination (see, for example, Debroy, 2020). It will be important for central and state government agencies to reflect on the lessons it has learned over the past year and ensure that these lessons inform policy deliberations going forward.

Foreign policy response

As India confirmed its first case of the novel coronavirus at the end of January 2020, it was hard to imagine the damage the virus would cause to India's economy and to its image as a rising power. With the number of COVID-19 cases growing slowly in India, the initial media focus was on China as the source of the problem. Since it was widely reported in the international media that the virus was first detected in Wuhan, the Indian media began to focus on the plight of Indians who were studying or working in China. As the disease was spreading rapidly in Wuhan and a grave situation emerging there, the news of the initial cover-up by the local Chinese authorities was also widely reported in the Indian media. However, as the Chinese government imposed a very strict lockdown in Wuhan and surrounding areas in late January and demonstrated its ability to quickly build new infrastructure to treat the coronavirus patients, including completing a new 1,000-bed hospital in a record ten days, the Indian public began to wonder how India would cope should the virus take hold in the country. As discussed above, India's public health care system is fragmented, and a large proportion of its population lacks access to basic healthcare despite improvements in recent years.

India's initial response to the outbreak of the virus in Wuhan was to offer sympathy and support to the people of China. In a video message posted on his Twitter account on 16 February, the Indian Ambassador to China, Vikram Misri, expressed his government's support for the Chinese people in their fight against the virus that had by then left more than 1,600 people dead in China. India also offered to do everything within its means to assist the people of China and promised to send a consignment of medical supplies to the country (Bhaya, 2020). A week earlier, Prime Minister Modi had written to President Xi Jinping of China, expressing his solidarity with the Chinese people and offering assistance. Subsequently, an Indian Air Force C-17 landed in Wuhan on 26 February 2020 with 15 tonnes of medical supplies, which were handed over to a local charity.

In the remainder of this section, we look at India's external response to the global health emergency by examining what we regard as the country's twin diplomatic objectives: (1) helping to craft a global policy response to the pandemic in order to avoid a major economic catastrophe with potentially serious domestic consequences; and (2) projecting India's image as a responsible regional and global power. It would become clear in the following discussion that Prime Minister Modi positioned himself at the centre of his government's efforts to achieve the above objectives. He sought to breathe new life into two organisations that he had in the past either ignored or considered irrelevant to advancing India's national interest – the South Asian Association for Regional Cooperation (SAARC) and the Non-Aligned Movement (NAM). But he also proactively engaged with the one organisation that he has found to be useful in promoting India's credentials as a rising power: The Group of Twenty (G-20), whose members 'account for 85% of the world economy, 75% of global trade, and two-thirds of the world's population' (Department of Foreign Affairs and Trade, 2020)

South Asian association for regional cooperation

Conscious of China's growing influence in India's immediate neighbourhood, the government was also keen to show that India was both willing and able to help its South Asian neighbours deal with the pandemic. On March 13, Prime Minister Modi tweeted: 'I would like to propose that the leadership of SAARC nations chalk out a strong strategy to fight Coronavirus. We could discuss, via video conferencing, ways to keep our citizens healthy. Together, we can set an example to the world, and contribute to a healthier planet.' (Modi, 2020a)

The response from South Asian countries was quick and generally favourable. Sri Lankan President Gotabaya Rajapaksa, Maldivian President Ibrahim Mohamed Solih, Nepalese Prime Minister K P Sharma Oli, Bhutanese premier Lotay Tshering, Bangladeshi Prime Minister Sheikh Hasina and the Afghan government, all welcomed the proposal. Two days later, on 15 March, a virtual summit meeting of SAARC leaders was held in response to Prime Minister Modi's call to develop a regional strategy to fight the virus. While most South Asian leaders attended the meeting, the prime minister of Pakistan did not, in what was described by a Pakistani newspaper as a 'calculated move to pre-empt Indian Prime Minister Narendra Modi's move to portray himself a leader spearheading the fight against coronavirus' (*The Tribune*, 2020). The SAARC Secretary-General and Sri Lankan diplomat, Esala Ruwan Weerakoon, also attended the virtual summit, aimed at sharing experiences and coordinating their response to the pandemic.

It is worth recalling here that SAARC, the body responsible for promoting regional cooperation among South Asian countries, had been paralysed for more than three-and-a-half years over tensions between India and Pakistan prior to the initiative by Prime Minister Modi to call a virtual meeting to respond to the coronavirus emergency. Its leaders have not formally met since the 18th SAARC Summit held in Kathmandu in November 2014. The 19th summit, which was to be held in Pakistan in 2016, was called off when India and several other member states refused to participate in the wake of a terrorist attack on an Indian military base in Kashmir, which India blamed on Pakistan-sponsored militants. These tensions were reflected in the decision by the Pakistan Prime Minister Imran Khan not to attend the virtual summit. Instead, the Pakistan PM deputised his Special Assistant on National Health Services, Zafar Mirza, to attend the virtual summit; Mirza then proceeded to raise the controversial bilateral issue of Jammu and Kashmir, which India regards as a taboo subject in regional and multilateral forums.

Regardless of the attempts by Pakistan to derail the process initiated by the Indian prime minister, India proposed the creation of a COVID-19 Emergency Fund and offered to make an initial contribution of US$10 million. Other South Asian countries also chipped in with Bangladesh pledging US$1.5 million, Nepal US$1 million, Afghanistan US$1 million, Sri

Lanka US$5 million, the Maldives US$200 thousand, and Bhutan US$100 thousand. After initial hesitation, Pakistan announced on 9 April that it would contribute US$3 million to the fund. Pakistan, however, insisted that regional efforts to fight the pandemic should be led by the SAARC secretariat, based in Kathmandu, and not India.

A series of meetings and workshops have taken place under the SAARC umbrella since the virtual summit in mid-March. India has also provided medicines, personal protective equipment (PPE) and food aid to other South Asian countries that needed them. For example, in a tweet on 20 April, the President of Afghanistan, Ashraf Ghani, thanked India for providing his country with 500,000 tablets of hydroxychloroquine, 100,000 tablets of paracetamol, and 75,000 metric tons of wheat (Ghani, 2020). India has also offered to keep on stand-by Rapid Response Teams of doctors and specialists, along with testing kits and other equipment, to be placed at the disposal of neighbouring countries, if required.

India organised a series of online training workshops for the emergency response teams of neighbouring countries, in which Pakistan again refused to participate. India has also offered to share with SAARC members the software behind its Integrated Disease Surveillance Portal to help trace possible virus carriers and the people they may have contacted.

India evacuated tens of thousands of its citizens who were stranded in China, the Middle East and other parts of the world following the imposition of lockdowns and travel restrictions by India and various other countries. Along with its own citizens, India also evacuated some of the citizens of the neighbouring countries, including Bangladesh, Maldives, Myanmar and Sri Lanka.

The ice broken by the SAARC initiatives to promote cooperation in tackling the pandemic has also paved the way for further high-level meetings of SAARC officials. In an informal virtual meeting of SAARC Foreign Ministers on the sidelines of the 75th session of the United Nations General Assembly, on 24 September, the External Affairs Minister of India, S. Jaishankar, reaffirmed India's commitment to its Neighbourhood First policy and 'towards building a connected, integrated, secure and prosperous South Asia' (*The Economic Times*, 2020). Jaishankar also pointed out that India has launched a COVID-19 Information Exchange Platform (COINEX) to facilitate exchange of specialised information. Among other initiatives supported by India was the development of a useful website by SAARC Disaster Management Centre to disseminate reliable information and updates on the evolving situation across SAARC member countries. SAARC Food Bank mechanism was also initiated to alleviate food shortages and other adverse impacts of the pandemic.

India's leadership in coordinating the South Asian response to COVID-19 drew praise from some world leaders. In an interview with an Indian news agency in May 2020, the Commonwealth Secretary-General Patricia Scotland said, 'people are looking to India for how Prime Minister Narendra Modi, the government and people of India have responded to the pandemic, controlled it and minimised it because it could have been so much worse' (*The New Indian Express*, 2020). She also said she was 'very impressed' with the way Prime Minister Modi pulled together the SAARC nations, including several Commonwealth members, to coordinate a response to the pandemic.

Non-aligned movement

When Prime Minister Modi chaired the SAARC leaders' virtual meeting on March 15, his cabinet colleague and trusted ally, Home Minister Amit Shah tweeted: 'with today's SAARC conference [the] world has witnessed the dawn of a new kind of diplomacy, which sets an example for the world to follow'. Shah also proclaimed that 'under Prime Minister Modi's leadership India will play a defining role towards solving global issues'. India under Modi has indeed tried to demonstrate to the world that it punches above its economic weight and that it is able and willing to be a responsible stakeholder in tackling global challenges.

Although India had of late given the Non-Aligned Movement (NAM), of which it is a co-founder, the cold shoulder – Modi skipped the 2016 and 2019 in-person NAM Summits, sending in his place the Vice President of India – yet, on 4 May 2020, the prime minister chose to attend the virtual summit of the NAM Contact Group to discuss the Movement's response to the COVID-19 pandemic. He told the summit, 'in the post-COVID world, we need a new template of globalization, based on fairness, equality, and humanity'. 'Despite our own needs, we have ensured medical supplies to over 123 partner countries, including 59 members of NAM' (Modi, 2020b).

In his address to the NAM virtual summit, Modi also said: 'We should develop a platform for all NAM countries, to pool our experiences, best practices, crisis-management protocols, research, and resources' (Shankar, 2020). He also did not miss the opportunity to take a dig at India's neighbour, Pakistan, when he said: 'Even as the world fights COVID-19, some people are busy spreading some other deadly viruses such as terrorism, fake news and doctored videos to divide communities and countries' (Modi, 2020b).

While Indian foreign policy has clearly moved away from the founding principles of the non-aligned movement as India develops closer security ties with the United States, Japan and Australia, India remains a NAM member. The Indian government is actively using all international platforms available to it to promote its image as a responsible stakeholder and using every possible opportunity to contrast itself with its neighbours, China and Pakistan. China's economy is roughly five times the size of India's and it provides more development assistance and makes more investments in developing countries, most of which are members of NAM, under its Belt and Road Initiative. But India prides itself on its softer, more friendly approach to other developing nations, which it contrasts with China's 'debt trap' diplomacy. If China is the 'factory of the world', Prime Minister Modi markets India as the 'pharmacy to the world' (*The Indian Express*, 2020).

G-20

The Indian prime minister was quick to pick up the phone and call other world leaders, offering India's help in combating the pandemic and appealing for greater global cooperation. Encouraged by his success in convening a virtual meeting of South Asian leaders to discuss their collective response to the pandemic, on 17 March Modi called the Saudi Crown Prince Mohammed bin Salman, the current G-20 chair, and suggested a virtual meeting of the world's 20 largest economies.

An 'extraordinary session' of the G-20 leaders was held on 26 March via video conference, at which Modi stressed the need to prioritise humanitarian interests in dealing with the pandemic. Earlier, in his telephone conversations with a number of world leaders, Modi had discussed his views on how the grouping could help coordinate its efforts in dealing with the pandemic. Among the leaders he spoke with were the British Prime Minister Boris Johnson and the Australian Prime Minister Scott Morrison, with whom he discussed the need for a G-20 meeting to plan a response to the virus. Separately, the Saudi government had said in a statement that,

> the G20 will act, alongside international organisations, in any way deemed necessary to alleviate the impact of the pandemic. G20 leaders will put forward a coordinated set of policies to protect people and safeguard the global economy. (Emirates News Agency, 2020)

The G-20 meeting resolved to 'fully support and commit to further strengthen the WHO's mandate in coordinating the international fight against the pandemic' and to 'close the financing gap' in the WHO Strategic Preparedness and Response Plan. The G-20 countries also said that they were collectively injecting US$5 trillion into the global economy as part of fiscal stimulus, economic measures and guarantee schemes (The G20, 2020).

When Modi proposed the idea of a G-20 summit to discuss a common response to the emerging pandemic, there were only 200,000 cases of COVID-19 infection worldwide and 8,200 people had died of the disease, according to the Johns Hopkins University Coronavirus Resource Center. Apparently, what drove Modi to call world leaders was the fear of a Global Financial Crisis-type of economic collapse in the wake of the pandemic. This would have dire consequences for the world economy, and it would also derail India's goal of becoming a US$5 trillion economy by 2025.

Critics have dubbed the Indian prime minister's enthusiastic early efforts to simultaneously combat the pandemic at home and position India as a leader in shaping global responses as 'Sisyphean' (Kugelman, 2020). India has indeed struggled to contain the spread of the virus at home and its diplomatic efforts to craft a global response to the pandemic have dissipated as it focuses its energies on managing the disease and its economic fallout. One reason for the loss of momentum is the fact that, faced with the pandemic, every country is trying to look after its own interests. India's scarce diplomatic and financial resources are currently stretched to the limit as it deals with a raging pandemic, slowing economy and an uncertain international environment, not to mention the heightened tensions along its border with China. Barely weeks after offering support and assistance to China in its fight against COVID-19, India had to contend with aggressive military manoeuvres by China along their disputed border in Ladakh in the Himalayas, leading to violent clashes and dozens of fatalities for the first time in decades. Though it is possible that the Chinese actions were designed to take advantage of the difficult situation confronting India in the face of the pandemic, it may be too early to determine the exact cause. Whatever the Chinese motivations, these dangerous manoeuvres have adversely affected Indian public opinion towards China, which had already soured following the alleged attempts by the Chinese authorities to conceal the novel coronavirus outbreak in Wuhan in December 2019.

Conclusion

This article has demonstrated how India is responding to the COVID-19 pandemic in both the domestic and international arenas. The health, economic and diplomatic policy challenges faced by India are enormous. But the economic growth of the past three decades has allowed India to cope with the policy challenges thrown up by the pandemic. India's domestic response to the global health emergency has been significant but stymied by weaknesses in policy coordination and social safety nets. For instance, the mass movement of migrant labour could have been prevented through more coordination with state and local governments, and labour market protections. However, these challenges are not new. Successive state and central governments have paid inadequate attention to addressing these fault lines. Though initially the prime minister relied heavily on his personal popularity to drive social and cultural changes necessary to contain the spread of the virus, this approach has been found wanting in the absence of a strong bureaucratic and nationally coordinated response to the pandemic. There has also been some evidence of policy learning and reflection on the experience across different states. For example, protocols of managing testing, quarantining, and even managing the illness are revised frequently (Sanyal, 2020). To the extent that these processes of learning are institutionalised, they will help in developing India's domestic capacity to deal with pandemics in the future.

In relation to foreign policy, India has taken bold initiatives at the regional and global levels to craft multilateral responses to the pandemic. It seized the initiative to lead a South Asian response to COVID-19 and demonstrate leadership at the global stage. The Indian government is using all available diplomatic platforms to project itself as a positive influence and responsible stakeholder in solving global problems. It has also made big strides as a trustworthy supplier of pharmaceuticals and personal protective equipment. But it faces a herculean task in trying to contain the spread of the virus at home pending the approval of an effective vaccine. Once that happens, as a leader in vaccine production, India would be in a good position to meet its domestic needs and supply the world with sufficient quantities of vaccines. But for the moment its international image has been dented by its inability to bring the spread of the virus under control and provide adequate levels of protection to the most vulnerable people in the country.

Acknowledgments

The authors would like to acknowledge research assistance by Surjeet Dhanji and thank the two anonymous reviewers for their valuable feedback.

Disclosure statement

No potential conflict of interest was reported by the authors.

References

Asher, M., Vora, Y., & Maurya, D. (2015). An analysis of selected pension and health care initiatives for informal sector workers in India. *Social Policy & Administration*, *49*(6), 738–751. https://doi.org/10.1111/spol.12167

Bajoria, R. (2020, November 12). *India: Fiscal announcements add to stimulus and deficit*. Barclays Research.

Bali, A. S., Capano, G., & Ramesh, M. (2019). Anticipating and designing for policy effectiveness. *Policy & Society*, *38*(1), 1–13. https://doi.org/10.1080/14494035.2019.1579502

Bali, A. S., & Ramesh, M. (2015). Health care reforms in India: Getting it wrong. *Public Policy and Administration*, *30*(3–4), 300–319. https://doi.org/10.1177/0952076715590697

Bardhan, P. (2020, May 21) *Modi's performance and the tragedy of India's poor*. Viewpoint. https://southasia.berkeley.edu/modi%E2%80%99s-performance-and-tragedy-india%E2%80%99s-poor
BBC. (2020, November 26). *India coronavirus: How do you vaccinate a billion people?* https://www.bbc.com/news/world-asia-india-55048925
Bhaya, A. (2020, February 16). *India pledges to send medical supplies to China in fight against novel coronavirus*. CGTN. https://news.cgtn.com/news/2020-02-16/India-pledges-medical-aid-to-China-in-fight-against-novel-coronavirus-O86odFe9P2/index.html
Business Today. (2020, September 20). *Nirmala takes opposition head-on over PM CARES fund*. https://www.businesstoday.in/current/economy-politics/nirmala-takes-opposition-head-on-over-pm-cares-fund/story/416533.html
Capano, G., Howlett, M., Jarvis, D. S., Ramesh, M., & Goyal, N. (2020). Mobilizing policy (in) capacity to fight COVID-19: Understanding variations in state responses. *Policy and Society, 39* (3), 285–308. https://doi.org/10.1080/14494035.2020.1787628
Centre for Internet and Society. (2020). *A survey of Covid 19 apps launched by state governments in India*. https://cis-india.org/internet-governance/stategovtcovidapps-pdf
Comptroller and Auditor General of India. (2019). *Press release on the audit report on GST tabled in Parliament*. Government of India. https://cag.gov.in/uploads/PressRelease/PR-Press-11-of-2019-05f5f6b0a3a6f39-81964485.pdf
Coronavirus Resource Centre. (2020). Johns Hopkins University. https://coronavirus.jhu.edu/map.html
Debroy, B. (2020). Seven governance issues raised by COVID. *Indian Public Policy Review, 1*(2), 16–25.
Department of Foreign Affairs and Trade. (2020). *The G20*. Government of Australia. https://www.dfat.gov.au/trade/organisations/g20/Pages/g20
DNA. (2020, October 20). *From March 19 to Oct 20, highlights of PM Modi's addresses to nation on COVID-19*. https://www.dnaindia.com/india/report-from-march-19-to-oct-20-highlights-of-pm-modi-s-speech-on-covid-19-2851154
Emirates News Agency. (2020, March 18). *Saudi Arabia calls for extraordinary 'virtual' G20 leaders' summit on coronavirus*. https://wam.ae/en/details/1395302831504
Financial Express. (2020, September 11). *Govt working on creating database of migrant labourers: Union minister Santosh Kumar Gangwar*. https://www.financialexpress.com/economy/govt-working-on-creating-database-of-migrant-labourers-union-minister-santosh-kumar-gangwar/2081020/
Ganpathy, N. (2020a February 5) Coronavirus: India starts screening passengers from Singapore. *Straits Times*. https://www.straitstimes.com/asia/south-asia/coronavirus-india-starts-screening-passengers-from-singapore
Ganpathy, N. (2020b. March 19). India bans incoming international flights for a week over virus. *Straits Times*. https://www.straitstimes.com/asia/south-asia/india-bars-international-commercial-passenger-flights-from-landing-in-country-for
Gettleman, J., & Schultz, K. (2020). Modi orders 3-week total lockdown for all 1.3 billion Indians. *New York Times*. https://www.nytimes.com/2020/03/24/world/asia/india-coronavirus-lockdown.html
Ghani, A. (2020, April 20). *Thank you my friend Prime Minister*. https://twitter.com/ashrafghani/status/1252203477016678400
Government of India. (2020, March 24). *Government of India issues orders prescribing lockdown for containment of COVID19 epidemic in the country*. New Delhi: Ministry of Home Affairs. https://pib.gov.in/PressReleaseIframePage.aspx?PRID=1607997
Kugelman, M. (2020, March 30). *Narendra Modi's Sisyphean quest for global coronavirus cooperation*. Foreign Policy. https://foreignpolicy.com/2020/03/30/narendra-modi-india-coronavirus-cooperation/
Mishra, A. R. (2020, March, 27) *Sitharaman announces ₹1.7 trillion package for the poor hit by the lockdown*. Live Mint. https://www.livemint.com/news/india/covid-19-centre-announces-rs-1-7-trillion-package-for-migrant-workers-poor-11585207289279.html

Modi, N. (2020a, March 13). *I would like to propose that the leadership of SAARC nations chalk out a strong strategy to fight Coronavirus.* Retrieved online from https://twitter.com/narendramodi/status/1238371182094639104?lang=en.

Modi, N. (2020b, May 4). *Intervention by the Prime Minister at the video conference of NAM contact group in response to COVID 19.* https://www.narendramodi.in/intervention-by-the-prime-minister-narendra-modi-at-video-conference-of-nam-contact-group-in-response-to-covid-19-549535

Nageswaran, V. A. (2020a, November 9). The train of structural reforms set in motion on Nov 8, 2016, has led to formalisation of the economy. *The Indian Express.* https://indianexpress.com/article/opinion/columns/demonetisation-india-economic-slowdown-gdp-data-covid-19-impact-7014835/

Nageswaran, V. A. (2020b, December 1) *Why it may be the wrong time to give up hope on India.* Swarajya. https://swarajyamag.com/economy/why-it-may-be-the-wrong-time-to-give-up-hope-on-india

Nature. (2020, September 3). *India will supply coronavirus vaccines to the world — Will its people benefit?* https://www.nature.com/articles/d41586-020-02507-x

Ramesh, M., & Bali, A. S. (2021). *Universal health care in Asia: A policy design approach.* Cambridge University Press. In press.

Ranjan, R. (2020). Impact of COVID-19 on migrant labourers of India and China. *Critical Sociology*, 089692052097507. https://doi.org/10.1177/0896920520975074

Ravi, A. (2020, April 21). Lockdown helped India but may spell economic doom: Shamika Ravi. *The New Indian Express.* https://www.newindianexpress.com/states/karnataka/2020/apr/21/interview–lockdown-helped-india-but-may-spell-economic-doom-shamika-ravi-2133004.html

Saha, M. (2020, October 9). RBI says GDP will contract by 9.5% in FY21, holds repo rate at 4% amid modest recovery. *The Print.*

Sanyal, S. (2020). Full conversation between New York Times journalist Suhasini Raj and Sanjeev Sanjyal. https://www.youtube.com/watch?v=u1FXfwrpcWE&feature=youtu.be

Sequeira, R. (2020, September 8). Taking over private hospitals for Covid-19 akin to nationalisation. *Times of India.* https://timesofindia.indiatimes.com/city/mumbai/taking-over-private-hospitals-for-covid-19-akin-to-nationalisation-maharashtra-govt-to-hc/articleshow/78000866.cms

Shankar, K. (2020, May 10). Modi reaches out to the world. The Statesman. https://www.thestatesman.com/opinion/modi-reaches-world-1502886596.html

The Economic Survey of India. (2017). *India on the move and churning: New evidence.* Government of India. https://www.indiabudget.gov.in/budget2017-2018/es2016-17/echap12.pdf

The Economic Times. (2020, December 6). *SAARC must deal with terrorism, obstruction in trade and connectivity: Jaishankar.* https://economictimes.indiatimes.com/news/politics-and-nation/saarc-must-deal-with-terrorism-obstruction-in-trade-and-connectivity-jaishankar/articleshow/78297226.cms

The Economic Times. (2020b, May 28). *3,736 Shramik Special trains ferried over 48 lakh migrants since May 1.* https://m.economictimes.com/industry/transportation/railways/3736-shramik-special-trains-ferried-over-48-lakh-migrants-since-may-1/articleshow/76074775.cms

The G20. (2020, March 26). *The G20 leaders statement.* https://reliefweb.int/sites/reliefweb.int/files/resources/G20_Extraordinary%20G20%20Leaders%E2%80%99%20Summit_Statement_EN%20%283%29.pdf19

The Hindu. (2020a, June 3). *Coronavirus | Setback for Arvind Kejriwal government's 'Delhi Corona' app.* The Hindu. https://www.thehindu.com/news/cities/Delhi/coronavirus-setback-for-arvind-kejriwal-governments-delhi-corona-app/article31743100.ece

The Hindu. (2020b, June 15). *60 lakh migrants took 4450 Sharmik specials to reach their home states.* https://www.thehindu.com/news/national/60-lakh-migrants-took-4450-shramik-specials-to-reach-their-home-states-railways/article31834747.ece

The Hindu. (2020c, December 13). *Coronavirus | India's COVID-19 cases per million among lowest in world.* https://www.thehindu.com/news/national/coronavirus-indias-covid-19-cases-per-million-among-lowest-in-world/article33319889.ece

The Indian Express. (2020, October 9). *PM Modi: India playing role of pharmacy to the world.* https://indianexpress.com/article/business/pm-modi-india-playing-role-of-pharmacy-to-the-world-6716524/
The New Indian Express. (2020, May 31). People look to India how PM Narendra Modi responded to COVID-19: Commonwealth Secretary-General Patricia Scotland.
The Tribune. (2020, April 9). Pakistan pledges $3m in SAARC COVID-19 Emergency Fund. https://tribune.com.pk/story/2194386/1-pakistan-pledges-3m-saarc-covid-19-emergency-fund
The Washington Post. (2020, November 11). *Who will make coronavirus vaccines for the developing world? India holds the key.* https://www.washingtonpost.com/world/asia_pacific/coronavirus-vaccine-india-serum-institute/2020/11/10/bbd7509c-0fb0-11eb-bfcf-b1893e2c51b4_story.html
The Wire. (2020, September 20). BJP dodges questions on accountability of PM-CARES Fund in Lok Sabha. https://thewire.in/government/pm-cares-fun-lok-sabha-bjp-congress-pmnrf
World Economic Forum. (2017, October 1). *India has 139 million internal migrants. They must not be forgotten.* https://www.weforum.org/agenda/2017/10/india-has-139-million-internal-migrants-we-must-not-forget-them/
Venkat, V. (2020, September 11) India: Why secrecy over Narendra Modi's coronavirus relief fund damages democracy. *The Conversation.* https://theconversation.com/india-why-secrecy-over-narendra-modis-coronavirus-relief-fund-damages-democracy-144897

COVID-19, Brexit and the United Kingdom – a year of uncertainty

Julie Smith

ABSTRACT
This article looks at the impact of the COVID-19 crisis in the United Kingdom. COVID-19 is a health issue but one that would have significant economic and constitutional implications for the UK. Moreover, the asymmetric responses across the UK put pressure on the very fabric of the country, as the four nations – Scotland, England, Wales and Northern Ireland – pursued differing policies in response to COVID-19 and within England certain regions perceived themselves to have been treated unfairly. All of these issues reinforced and magnified the implications of the issue that had overshadowed British politics for years: Brexit.

Introduction

'Europe shuts door on Britain over fears of mutant virus' ran a headline in December 2020, thereby aptly summarising the predicament in which the UK found itself as leaders sought to tackle a pandemic and the tortuous path out of the European Union (EU) (see Clatworthy et al., 2020). The COVID-19 (hereinafter referred to as 'COVID') pandemic hit the UK just as it officially left the European Union. January 2020 was the time for the UK to focus on forging a new relationship with the EU27 after four years during which the hotly contested topic of 'Brexit' had dominated political debate and, for advocates of Brexit at least, the time to 'go global'.[1] Such expectations were overturned or at least stalled by the unexpected and overwhelming impact of a global pandemic. The British Government's reaction was slow,[2] leading to some of the worst health outcomes globally during the first wave, despite a focus on protecting the National Health Service (NHS) and saving lives.[3] When it came, the Government's response was dramatic in terms of the economic consequences of lockdown and verged on the draconian in the sweeping powers it sought to deploy, minimising the role of Parliament and leading to concerns that liberty and democracy were dying (Forsyth, 2020a; Sumption, 2020).

This article looks at the impact of the COVID crisis on British politics and the economy, highlighting the unequal effects of COVID and the public policy responses to it across the United Kingdom. It argues that the unprecedented economic decisions taken, without adequate scrutiny, will have long-term consequences for the UK, as decades of fiscal prudence were cast aside in an attempt to minimise unemployment and ensure that people would obey the new rules imposed almost overnight on 26 March, encapsulated in the slogan: Stay Home; Protect the NHS; Save Lives. Moreover, the asymmetric responses across the UK put pressure on the very fabric of the country, as the four nations – Scotland, England, Wales and Northern Ireland – pursued differing policies in response to COVID and within England certain regions perceived themselves to be treated unfairly. COVID was a health issue but one that would have significant economic and constitutional implications for the UK. All of these issues reinforced and magnified the implications of the issue that had overshadowed British politics for years: Brexit. We turn first to the Coronavirus Act 2020 before looking at the implications of the policy choices made for health outcomes, the economy, education and the constitutional order of the United Kingdom.

The Coronavirus Act 2020 – government by executive fiat?

The British Government initially favoured responding to COVID via the creation of 'herd immunity' as practised until late 2020 by Sweden (see Colfer, 2020). By mid-March, however, the Government began to adopt an approach similar to that of other states, encouraging people to stay at home and work from home, and eventually ordering a complete lockdown. Less bureaucratic than, say, France where people had to have written documentation if they wished to leave their homes during lockdown, the British version nonetheless posed an unprecedented challenge to people's personal freedoms, notably any rights to free association, as the numbers of people permitted to meet together was capped at six (except for households larger than six).

Introducing the initial primary legislation to deal with the COVID crisis, the Secretary of State for Health, Matt Hancock (2020, col. 35), stated that 'Coronavirus is the most serious public health emergency that has faced the world in a century.' Thus 'To defeat it, *we are proposing extraordinary measures of a kind never seen before in peacetime*. Our goal is to protect life and to protect every part of the NHS' (emphasis added). That 'extraordinary measures' were required few doubted but the extent of the powers and their legal basis came under challenge – to a limited extent at the outset of the crisis, more vocally in late 2020 as renewed restrictions were repeatedly imposed and extended in England.[4] On 19 December 2020, just six days before a long-promised relaxation of the rules for a five-day period over Christmas, the Prime Minister held a press conference to announce that the health situation had deteriorated so significantly that new rules would be imposed by midnight that day – MPs from his own party complained about their inability to scrutinise the new legal measures, only to told that they could vote on them in January 2021, long after they had come into effect.[5] This was part of a pattern.

Continuing a practice pursued by Boris Johnson as he attempted to 'get Brexit done' (Smith, forthcoming 2021), the COVID crisis saw HMG seeking to minimise the role of Parliament as it sought emergency powers to tackle the crisis. The 342-page Coronavirus Act 2020 was passed at breath-taking speed, completing all stages in the House of Commons in a single day. Quite how any MP could have read and analysed the content of the Bill before it was debated and voted upon is unclear. There was certainly no time for detailed scrutiny of the legislation. True, the emerging health situation was deemed an emergency but the extent of the legislation and its impact on civil liberties was significant. Moreover, the legislation was originally intended to last for two years until former Cabinet Minister, Conservative MP David Davis called for a review after six months. The Government itself put forward an amendment for such a review (Hancock, 2020). Such a vote, however, would be on the continuation of the Act on a take-it-or-leave-it basis, not providing MPs with an opportunity to amend parts of the legislation that had proved not to work or which could be viewed as disproportionate.

Moreover, in the intervening six months many changes to government policy would be introduced with little or no scrutiny – further constraints on people's freedoms were introduced via statutory instruments (SIs) that were frequently debated long after they had come into effect (Forsyth, 2020a) and which were not subject to amendment (Forsyth, 2020b). The inability of Parliament to amend the legislation was a consequence of the Government's choice of legislative procedures, which provided wide powers for executive action: SIs are not amendable, unlike primary legislation, meaning MPs and peers were faced with 'take-it-or-leave' choices on mechanisms to try to tackle the crisis. Few wished to thwart the Government's actions entirely but over time they became increasingly frustrated at the extension of provisions brought forward without any impact assessment being provided (see *Hansard*, 4 November 2020). As Ronan Cormacain of the British Institute of International and Comparative Law told the House of Commons Public Administration and Constitutional Affairs Committee (2020, Question 10):

> The Coronavirus Act made a lot of changes but *a lot of the detailed social distancing rules, the lockdown rules, are being done by secondary legislation.* The clear distinction is that an Act of Parliament is something that you will see, debate, scrutinise and amend. The secondary legislation does not have that same level of parliamentary scrutiny. It is essentially for you to assent or disagree with but there is nothing more to it than that (emphasis added).

That the Government could propose its regulations, including the initial lockdown rules in March 2020 and again in November 2020,[6] in a way that offered Parliament so little time to scrutinise them arose from the fact that the Government opted to legislate within the provisions of the Public Health (Control of Diseases) Act 1984 rather than the Civil Contingencies Act (CCA) 2004. As former Supreme Court Justice Lord Sumption (2020) points out, the latter Act 'is the only statute specifically designed for emergencies serious enough to require the kind of measures that we have had. It authorises ministers to make regulations to deal with a wide variety of "events or situations", including those which threaten "serious damage to human welfare" … In other words it authorises government by executive decree.' The Public Health (Control of Diseases) Act 1984 does not envisage such wide-ranging powers, or 'executive fiat' as former Commons Speaker Bercow (2020) deemed it, since it applies to the sick, not the whole society. Yet the CCA provides for far more detailed parliamentary scrutiny than the Health Act; scrutiny to which the Government seemed unwilling to subject itself.

By certifying the Coronavirus Bill to be a 'money bill', the Speaker of the House of Commons ensured that the House of Lords would not play a part in enacting that significant piece of primary legislation.[7] Occasionally the decision that draft legislation should be deemed a 'money bill' can seem like a ruse to avoid peers playing a significant role, particularly if they appear to be at odds with the will of the elected house, since the lack of a majority for any party in the upper house means that governments of whatever political complexion cannot assume their legislative proposals will get through unamended. However, in the case of the Coronavirus Act as enacted there could be little doubt that 'money' was involved. The Queen signalled her agreement that 'for the purposes of any Act arising from the Coronavirus Bill, it is expedient to authorise the payment of money provided by Parliament of –

(a) any expenditure which is incurred by a Minister of the Crown, government department or any other public authority by virtue of this Act,
(b) any increase attributable to this Act in the sums payable by virtue of any other Act out of money so provided, and
(c) any other expenditure which is incurred (whether before or after the passing of this Act) by a Minister of the Crown, government department or other public authority in connection with the making of payments, or the giving of financial assistance to a person (whether directly or indirectly), as a result of coronavirus or coronavirus disease' (*Hansard*, 674, 23 March 2020).

This declaration of a money bill is a routine practice, yet it is worth reproducing in its entirety precisely because of the scope of the Coronavirus Act 2020 and the enormity of the financial commitments made by the Prime Minister and his Chancellor of Exchequer and the associated Contingencies Fund Act enacted on the same day. Over the course of the next eight months the Chancellor would make repeated statements designed to reassure businesses and individuals, making hundreds of billions of pounds' worth of pledges, as discussed in the next section. This was no mere pro-forma commitment to spending but rather the start of a series of expensive commitments that would potentially impact the UK economy for generations as a result inter alia of 'the highest recorded level of borrowing in our peacetime history' (Sunak, 2020).

Parliamentary scrutiny was further limited by the need to review working arrangements for both houses, given the very confined spaces in both the Lords and Commons chambers, so different from more modern parliamentary buildings including the European Parliament, *bête noire* of Brexiteers, where MPs have their own dedicated desks, microphones and sufficient space to be 'socially distanced,' to use the rather bizarre term that became a key part of the English language during 2020, far less provision for electronic voting. Thus, there were initially some changes that ensured MPs and peers' ability to scrutinise the government would be minimised both because of long recesses and foreshortened working hours and because the number of spaces available for members to sit was dramatically reduced to enable 'social distancing'. The House of Commons voted through the Coronavirus Act 2020 and immediately went into Recess. This coincided with the start of the first lockdown but since one of the exceptions to lockdown related to those who could not work from home, it would have been possible for the Commons to meet, given the absence of remote working facilities. The failure of MPs to do so led former President of the Supreme Court Lady (Brenda) Hale to rail against Parliament for surrendering 'control to the government at a crucial time' (Lady Hale as cited in Bowcott et al., 2020).

The House of Lords was apprised of the timetable for the Coronavirus Bill and the Contingencies Fund Bill by the Leader of the House, Baroness Evans, and promptly went into a four-week Recess. The arrangements for the Lords on their return saw the scope for debate and scrutiny much reduced as sitting times were cut to three short days a week. The situation was compounded by the fact that members of the Lords, like everyone else were subject to the rules of the lockdown, which required the over-70s to stay at home –

since the average age of peers is around 70, this meant many could not attend. Traditionally, there has been no possibility for MPs or peers to work remotely, no right to proxy voting and, as noted, no electronic voting. The Commons swiftly adopted remote working, while the Lords took somewhat longer to develop a hybrid system combining in-person and virtual attendance.

The Leader of the House of Commons, Jacob Rees-Mogg, soon insisted that MPs should return to their place of work, leading by example in attending the workplace, despite the fact that the Government's message was that people should work from home where they could. Having just trialled virtual proceedings, MPs had proved that they could indeed work from home. This was just one of the myriad examples of the Government sending mixed messages, contributing to confusion across the country, which would only be exacerbated as the Government tried to loosen lockdown arrangements of the summer and then re-impose them in the autumn. In line with the confused and inconsistent messages to the general public, parliamentarians were initially encouraged to stay at home and then encouraged to attend Parliament in person. Eventually, the Lords were to settle for the hybrid system, with remote voting the only way to cast a vote. The model could be seen as satisficing rather than wholly satisfactory as glitches in the technology at times led to votes having to be re-run and amendments not being moved as the 'virtual' peer could not be seen or heard. The situation was scarcely conducive to effective scrutiny of the Government's political, health or economic decisions: decisions consistently came several days or even weeks after the medical advice was to act.

Balancing health and the economy

COVID was first and foremost a health emergency but one with wide-ranging implications *inter alia* for personal liberties, international and domestic travel, and – especially – for the economy (see HM Treasury 2020). The profound changes wrought by the pandemic on lives and livelihoods arising from the need to lockdown in order to try to stem transmission of the virus led to dramatic economic changes and state intervention of a sort previously inconceivable under a Conservative administration. Coming at the end of winter when there was already seasonal pressure on hospital beds, the arrival of COVID-19 created a potential health and healthcare crisis in the UK. It was essential to try to reduce infection rates and, hence, hospital admissions and potentially deaths.

The Government initially treated the matter as a health issue, with Secretary of State for Health Matt Hancock playing a large role in fronting the policies. The capacity of the NHS to cope with this new challenge formed a crucial part of policy-making, with the Government stressing the importance of 'saving the NHS', apparently as an end in itself rather than for the health benefits it provides. The focus on the NHS was reminiscent of the suggestions during the 2016 referendum on EU membership that it would be better to send £350 million a week to the NHS than to the EU.[8] It gained traction and the message seemed to work: the first lockdown saw people stay at home as the law demanded – but come to their doors to clap the NHS workers every Thursday evening. Cynics might have thought that putting more money into the NHS and ensuring that there were sufficient medical personnel to staff the newly erected Nightingale hospitals established to deal with mass hospitalisations that never arose during the first wave would have been more beneficial to the healthcare sector. In practice the hospitals lacked the staff and were not used in the first wave; as a second wave emerged in Autumn 2020 frustrated MPs began to ask why the emergency hospitals could not be used rather than reverting to national lockdowns but the lack of medical personnel remained an issue.

There was a need to stop the transmission of the virus. Hence, the Coronavirus Act 2020 and the Government's decision to make the whole country go into lockdown from 26 March. This unprecedented requirement in a peacetime context was deemed necessary to avoid mass fatalities and ensure the NHS did not collapse – a key concern for the Prime Minister as the country prepared for a second lockdown in November 2020 (Johnson, 2020). Yet, closing schools, universities, businesses and places of worship, while also 'pausing' routine operations, would have major, long-term consequences for the mental and physical health of people in the UK as well as for the economy. Routine medical procedures and testing were dramatically reduced, although they did not cease entirely (NHS Providers, 2020), and non-emergency dental work cancelled; aside from growing waiting times for routine operations, there was a significant increase in mental health referrals (up 4.7% between March and June 2020), while 'Anecdotally [NHS] trusts report significant increases in demand for early intervention services, often linked to the wider impacts of COVID-19 such as economic hardship' (NHS Providers, 2020, p. 2). Decisions were announced piecemeal, with announcements on the COVID-related health matters coming first before the Government gave any indication of whether or how it would mitigate the effects of effectively shutting down the country.

The newly-minted Chancellor of the Exchequer,[9] Rishi Sunak, who had only assumed that role in February 2020, started to make a series of well-received announcements, initially relating to 'furlough' – a word almost unknown before March 2020 although similar policies were introduced in other European countries in response to COVID (see House of Lords Economic Affairs Committee, 2020, p. 15). The proposal was to allow furloughed workers to receive 80% of pay if they were unable to work during the lockdown, paid for by the Government. In some cases, employers would top up their pay to 100%. Thus, for some employees there was security of income without the requirement to work. Most parents were required to educate their children at home, while furloughed or, perhaps most stressful of all, while working full-time from home. Little thought was given to whether households had the space or resources to home educate their children, whose prospects would be impeded by lack of computers and high-speed broadband. Schools did remain open for the children of key workers, including healthcare workers and teachers, but the provision was not extended to children whose families could not manage to teach them. Whether individuals who were furloughed would have jobs to return to after the end of lock-down was unclear, but the short-term impact of the policy was clear and effective; to avoid mass unemployment.

This was a marked change of direction from a party which in the 1980s had considered unemployment 'a price worth paying' for tackling what it perceived as the scourge of inflation. Day after day Sunak came forward with new initiatives – and new money – to deal with the increasing numbers of special cases that were emerging. The budget was pushed into the long grass and a multi-annual review was instead to be just a one-year review, set for late November 2021. The policies initially seemed un-costed and the consequences would fall on subsequent generations of taxpayers, themes that were repeatedly raised with Ministers, but rarely elicited a clear answer. In the short-term however, the Chancellor met the objective of saving jobs; unemployment began to rise but not exponentially (see Brewer et al., 2020) as 8.9 million jobs were supported by the Job Retention Scheme at its height in April 2020 (House of Lords Economic Affairs Committee, 2020, p. 10). In November 2020 the Office of Budgetary Responsibility would predict that unemployment was likely to peak at 7.5% or 2.6 million people in the second quarter of 2021 once the Job Retention Schemed ended – high but not unprecedented and lower than the figures in some other European countries (Office for Budget Responsibility, 2020; see also House of Lords Economic Affairs Committee, 2020, p. 11).

Nonetheless, the impact of COVID and its economic consequences would affect different strands of society differently. As the Chancellor pointed out in his 2020 Spending Review, the wages of public sector workers rose while those in the private sector fell (see Sunak 2020). Meanwhile, the self-employed did not receive such generous treatment from the Government's Job Retention Scheme (the original scheme for furlough, later renamed the Job Support Scheme) as businesses, and such funding as there was for the self-employed was poorly targeted (House of Lords Economic Affairs Committee, 2020, p. 21). The Resolution Foundation found that at the peak of the crisis in April 2020, 30% of the self-employed had no pay; the figure for employees was 4% (Brewer et al., 2020, p. 57). Free-lancers, especially in the arts and creative industries found themselves in a precarious situation, while paradoxically those in the gig economy saw their income increase dramatically as shoppers switched online and diners used delivery services.

Aside from keeping businesses afloat and paying wages, the Chancellor also sought to ensure people kept a roof over their head by allowing mortgage repayments to be frozen. Landlords were also temporarily prevented from evicting tenants during the crisis. And then, in an attempt to stimulate the hospitality sector as the UK emerged from its first lock-down, the 'eat out to help out' scheme began, offering half-price restaurant meals during August. The idea was simultaneously to encourage people to socialise again and, especially, to spend money, after the immense success of the 'stay home' slogan left people reluctant to resume anything like their normal lives (Hope & Dixon, 2020). The scheme was a success by some measures: 161,934,000 meals were claimed from 3 to 31 August (House of Commons Library, 2020a, p. 13). Yet, by other measures, it could be seen as encouraging people to socialise too closely, contributing to the resurgence of COVID transmissions in Autumn 2020. The original message to stay home had been clear, as were the rules of the lockdown.

As the UK emerged from lockdown, the new messages were more muddled – 'stay alert; stop the virus' might have sounded alliterative but it was imprecise and vague: how being alert could stop an invisible killer was unclear. Nonetheless, from the Chancellor's perspective, the eat-out-to-help-out scheme had delivered. Moreover, Sunak saw his popularity sky-rocket, above that of the Prime Minister – possibly the only British politician to see their star in the ascendant at this time.[10] The total cost of Sunak's beneficence was £280 billion in 2020, leading to predicted Government borrowing of £394 billion for the year, representing almost 20% of GDP or, as Sunak himself put it, 'The highest recorded level of borrowing in our peacetime history' (Sunak, 2020).

Beyond the financing of the crisis response, a range of societal issues arose that ensured that the crisis would hit some people more than others. They ranged from the impact of COVID itself through other health-related matters, including mental health and, especially, education. As schools closed their doors for months on end, parents were expected to 'home school' their children while simultaneously working from home. Such a situation might have been feasible for families with the resources to have desks, stable broadband facilities and the time to educate their children while working flexibly from home themselves. Yet, as with so many issues associated with COVID, educational inequalities were compounded during lockdown as some schools were able to offer effective remote teaching while others were less able to do so. Family and financial situations meant that the knock-on effects of lockdown would persist through the examination period and into university admissions, which proved chaotic, as the Government made one U-turn after another regarding whether schools should or should not open and whether examinations would be taken or not. When and whether schools could re-open and in what form depended, like so many of the COVID responses, on which part of the UK one lived in.

A (dis)United Kingdom

Responses to the crisis differed across the United Kingdom, further highlighting the impact of twenty years of devolution on the fabric of the Union. While the Coronavirus Act 2020 covers the whole of the UK, various aspects of policy formation and delivery are devolved to the nations, namely Scotland, Wales and Northern Ireland – this includes public health (Colfer, 2020, p. 208). Thus, rather than a single 'united' response to COVID, the Prime Minister's pronouncements in London were not always replicated in Edinburgh, Cardiff and Belfast. Daily press conferences in London led by the PM or a Cabinet minister plus leading scientific and medical advisors were matched by televised daily briefings from Scottish First Minister Nicola Sturgeon, until BBC Scotland eventually stopped showing Sturgeon's briefings. While the BBC explained the change as the result of the Scottish Parliament returning to business as usual (BBC News, 2020), the assumption was that they were dropped because they gave the First Minister too much (positive) coverage, compared to the PM. The BBC reported that Scottish Conservatives had 'claimed Nicola Sturgeon had at times used the daily briefings as a political platform to criticise the UK government' (BBC News 2020). This seemingly minor issue is nonetheless indicative of growing tensions in the UK over the role of the main public service broadcaster.

It was not merely in presentational matters that the leaders of the four nations came into conflict. By the autumn of 2020, they were each taking markedly different decisions over renewed lockdowns and whether or not to move to national rather than localised lockdowns. In Scotland, a 'five-level system of COVID-19 restrictions' was approved by the Scottish Parliament on 27 October, resulting in different arrangements across Scotland according to infection levels (BBC Scotland News, 2020). Wales was the first to change tack with First Minister Mark Drakeford announcing a 17-day national lockdown – or what he called 'a firebreak' – in Wales from 23 October until 9 November. Like Wales, Northern Ireland (NI) also moved to lockdown. Its decision was swiftly followed' before by the decision taken in Dublin that the Republic of Ireland would go into a second lockdown. This local situation highlighted and foreshadowed a much wider challenge for the United Kingdom as it prepared, however invisibly, for Brexit, namely, the twin relationships of Northern Ireland with Great Britain and with the Republic, which remains a member of the EU. Northern Ireland went into a second lockdown on

16 October and pledged to come out of it on 13 November, regardless of what happened in the England. Moreover, the restrictions in NI were rather looser than in England even under lockdown conditions (see NI Direct, 2020). The different reactions reflected not so much different incidences of the virus, so much as different policy choices (Colfer, 2020). The effect was to reinforce wider national differences and raise the spectre of the break-up of the United Kingdom.

Yet it was not only the devolved nations that sought to disagree with the Government's responses to COVID. The effects of the disease and the policies adopted to try to tackle it had differential impacts in different parts of England, with those parts of the North of England that had voted for the Conservatives to 'get Brexit done' in 2019 among the worst affected. Where the PM's erstwhile Special Advisor had pressed for a 'levelling up' to support those regions, the reality seemed like a levelling down. Rather than consider the epidemiology the emphasis from regional leaders, typically elected mayors such as the Mayor of Manchester, former Labour MP Andy Burnham, seemed to focus heavily on 'fairness'.

Thus, even within England, the Government's response to COVID caused profound tensions. Having relaxed the first lockdown very gradually over the summer, the PM was determined to avoid a second national lockdown – a battle as already noted that he lost on 31 October. As Kuenssberg (2020) put it: 'Nuclear weapon. Misery. Disaster. That's what he called it. And yet that is what he has done.' Prior to this renewed nuclear option, a series of restrictions were in place, including the 'rule of six', under which up to six people could meet indoors. In England children were included in the limit, whereas in Scotland for a similar rule they were not, leading to frustration in England; why should children pose a risk in England but not Scotland, one wondered. In a federal country, such different policy choices might be seen as a normal fact of political life. The UK with its asymmetric devolution in which decision-making in England remains highly centralised, it created significant political sensitivity. Public health decisions including on the essential test, track and trace were taken centrally rather than devolved to people with local knowledge such as local health authorities, as were decisions on procurement of vital equipment, including personal protective equipment and ventilators. This would lead to controversy as contracts were handed to people and businesses with little experience but, allegedly, close contacts with the Conservative Party. Thus, the *New York Times* conducted an investigation into cronyism (Bradley et al., 2020), while the National Audit Office (2020) noted that £10.5 billion of the contracts for goods and services by value (out of £17.5 billion) were let without competition.

As the numbers of COVID cases began to rise again, particularly in the North East and North West of England, the Government had attempted to create a three-tier system that would enable more stringent restrictions to be imposed in areas with very high levels of infection (Tier 3) and high levels of infection (Tier 2) than were required in 'medium' areas (Tier 1). (Nowhere in the country was deemed to have 'low' rates of infection by the time the Tiers were introduced.) As with the earlier national lock-down, there was little time for Parliament to scrutinise the additional restrictions imposed. The necessary Statutory Instruments were debated in the House of Lords on the day they had become law. The government determined which local areas would be moved into the higher tiers, following negotiations with leaders of the local authorities and/or directly elected mayors. One of the key issues for local leaders was to secure funding for their cities or regions to try to offset some of the financial consequences of the renewed restrictions. The Government decided that tighter rules were necessary in one particular area: the Liverpool City Region, which went into Tier Three measures in mid-October. While the PM believed that Greater Manchester should similarly be subject to Tier Three restrictions, these were delayed as a result of protracted negotiations with the Mayor, Andy Burnham, who held out, ultimately unsuccessfully, for more money for his region. The Prime Minister found himself unexpectedly engaged in two sets of negotiations by mid-October, with leaders of the English regions and with the EU, reflecting the UK's changing constitutional order towards greater national devolution and an attempt to return powers from the EU. Such negotiations would persist, limiting the PM's capacity to focus on either COVID or Brexit.

Brexit

Political debate had turned overnight from Brexit to COVID in March. The UK's departure from the EU was negotiated in such a way that although the resultant Withdrawal Agreement ensured the UK's formal departure on 31 January 2020, for an eleven-month transitional period the UK was to continue to enjoy many of the benefits of normally associated with membership in return for abiding by the rules – and contributing to the EU budget. During this period, the EU and UK were due to negotiate their future relationship – the shape of which remained unclear almost four years after the referendum. Red lines proposed by Theresa May in 2018 and reinforced by Boris Johnson ensured that models of close cooperation such as membership of the European Economic Area alongside Norway, Iceland and Liechtenstein were not an option for the UK. The EU was reluctant to have a series of bespoke bilateral agreements along the lines Switzerland had negotiated over decades.

Thus, it seemed that two Commonwealth countries offered examples for the future relationship – Canada, with its Comprehensive Economic and Trade Agreement with the European Union (CETA) and Australia, which leading Conservative Brexiteers began to advocate as a model for UK-EU relations, despite not having a comprehensive Free Trade Agreement with the EU, its relations being based on a network of agreements (Murray & Matera, 2020), including a 'framework agreement' (Bevington, 2020). Slightly better than trading on World Trade Organization (WTO) terms, the 'Australia model' would still have offered UK businesses very limited benefits compared with membership of the internal market. Indeed, former Australian PM Malcolm Turnbull, told the UK to 'be careful what you wish for', stating that 'Australians wouldn't regard our trade relationship with Europe as a satisfactory one' (as cited in Morris, 2020). Whereas the WTO arrangements might allow tariff-free trade, they do not in any way begin to replicate the non-tariff barrier arrangements that the UK enjoyed as a member of the European Union. Such was the agenda as the UK and its European neighbours ended 2020.

The Brexit issues did not go away during the COVID crisis but they did slip down the political agenda, despite the fact that the clock continued to tick towards the end of the transition period on 31 December 2020, which would mark the final stage of departure from the EU. It was a date that the Prime Minister refused to extend, despite the difficulty of conducting the negotiations at the height of the pandemic, and the need to complete the negotiations in sufficient time for any future trade deal to be ratified by the European Parliament and, depending on the nature of such an agreement, potentially also national parliaments. In March 2020 all the key negotiators suffered from COVID and face-to-face meetings were cancelled. By the end of the year, virtual meetings had become a fact of life for politicians and civil servants as for everyone else. When the pandemic first hit, arrangements were not in place for such remote working.

Gradually, negotiations were reconvened virtually but such encounters lack one of the crucial features of normal EU negotiations – the side or 'corridor' conversations, the informal meetings in the margins of the formal discussions which can help to forge solutions and also assist negotiators in getting to know their interlocutors. Arguably by March 2020 the key actors already knew each other rather well. Nonetheless, the dynamics shifted and discussions appeared to falter. They eventually resumed in person but progress was slow. Despite the Prime Minister's insistence that the negotiations could not continue beyond the mid-October meeting of the European Council, which would make the final decision on the future relationship on behalf of the EU, negotiations continued on into November and then December. Indeed, on 16 October, the day after Johnson hoped the matter would have finally been resolved, he found himself in negotiations with both the EU27 and with the elected mayors of various Northern cities. This was scarcely the scenario he had planned when he romped home at the polls in the December 2019 general election barely ten months earlier on the platform: Get Brexit Done.

Rather, he was seeking to ensure that a further national (England-wide) lockdown could be avoided. Yet within two weeks new rumours emerged that a national lockdown was on the cards; a month after the scientific evidence had suggested that a 'circuit-breaker' would be necessary. At that stage the PM was trying to avert another economically damaging lockdown. Hence, the rather complex tier-system. Claiming that there had been a leak, the PM hastily convened a press conference on Halloween at which he announced that there would indeed be a further period of lock-down, arguing 'Now is the time because there is no alternative' (Johnson, 2020). The earlier rhetoric of 'Stay home; save lives; protect the NHS' was dusted down and reused. Four days later the relevant legislation had been passed in Parliament, paving the way for a four-week period of lockdown in England, just days before Wales was due to end its firebreak. That the four nations of the United Kingdom were taking different approaches could have reflected the epidemiology; differing rates of infection could plausibly have made differing responses appropriate. However, the effect was to make it difficult for citizens of the UK to move between the four nations, even if parts of the country were not officially locked down.

One point of agreement was that the four nations should follow similar rules over the Christmas period. The PM and three First Ministers agreed to a five-day relaxation of the rules, allowing three households or 'bubbles' to come together between the 23 and 27 December regardless of which nation or region people came from. Plans were made accordingly, but a week before Christmas plans were derailed as the rates of infection began to soar. London and parts of the South and East of England were put into a new Tier Four, banned from travelling over the Christmas period. The Scottish First Minister announced that people would not be able to travel between England and Scotland. It appeared that the PM's nightmare was being played out: he would have to thwart people's Christmas plans. For the leader of the Opposition, this was simply yet another case of the right decision being made far too late – Keir Starmer had, after all, repeatedly called for the Government to act on the basis of the advice it was receiving from the Scientific Advisory Group on Emergencies (SAGE), only to be rebuffed before a prime ministerial volte-face just days late, but critically late in terms of responding to the crisis. It quickly transpired that the UK was the source of a new, mutant version of COVID-19, which spread faster than the original: the decision to curtail Christmas plans domestically was thus rapidly augmented by the decisions of EU states (and many others beside) to ban flights from the UK – Christmas seemed to be cancelled and the country that sought to be free of the EU was now excluded from it by a virus.

Conclusions

Coupled with Brexit, the COVID crisis impacted the UK in a variety of ways. The fact that the four nations had different responses to the crisis highlights yet again the impact of devolved government on the United Kingdom itself. That Nicola Sturgeon appeared to be handling the crisis rather better than Boris Johnson gave further impetus to those seeking Scottish independence; elections to the devolved assemblies are due in May 2021 after a year-long postponement because of the pandemic, itself a further indication of the impact of the COVID crisis on democratic practices in the UK. Scotland may not have performed better than England in health outcomes, but Sturgeon handled the PR side of things far more effectively. Boris Johnson, for all he might have acquired draconian powers, seemed unable to make key decisions in a timely way. Rather, the experience of COVID – both as a national crisis and as a personal health issue that saw him hospitalised with COVID in March 2020 — led the PM to recognise the need to stop COVID but conflicted as his colleagues railed against decisions than would inevitably have serious, long-term consequences for the economy.

The upshot was a series of reluctantly taken decisions that were made too late if one listened to the medical evidence. Consequently, by the time decisions were reached they were more significant and, hence, more controversial than if a modest decision had been taken in more timely fashion. The UK thus ended 2020 divided, impoverished and more unequal that it had begun. What was hoped to be a short-term crisis looked set to have long-term consequences at home and knock-on consequences for the UK's relations with the EU. A PM who sought to take back control faced a toxic combination of Brexit (unresolved) and COVID-mutant variant (uncontrolled), leading to flights being banned and Calais closed to lorries. True, the UK and EU did finally come to terms on their future relationship in the guise of the EU-UK Trade and Cooperation Agreement on 24 December 2020. However, an unseemly scramble to secure COVID vaccines in early 2021 demonstrated just how far relations between the erstwhile partners had deteriorated.

Notes

1. Article 50 of the Treaty on European Union indicates that a Withdrawal Agreement should be negotiated taking the future relationship between the EU and the withdrawing state into consideration. However, the EU-27 insisted that the negotiations for departure and the future relationship should be undertaken sequentially rather than in parallel. As discussed below, this ensured that at the height of the COVID crisis, the British Government was seeking simultaneously to tackle COVID and negotiate the future relationship, which would prove challenging for the Government.
2. Colfer (2020) highlights how much faster Ireland responded to cases than the UK, for example.
3. When the pandemic started, virologists predicted a second wave of the virus would occur; at the time of writing Europe was at the epicentre of the second wave. The present article

focuses primarily on the first wave in order to provide a degree of analysis beyond the purely transient and journalistic.

4. While the initial lockdown that started on 26 March was UK wide, covering all four nations, subsequent arrangements were increasingly made at a national level, sometimes co-ordinated between Prime Minister and the First Ministers of the Devolved Administrations, sometimes not.
5. Reflecting the frustration of many MPs, Charles Walker, the Deputy Chair of the 1922 Committee, which brings together backbench Conservative MPs, railed against the decision not to recall Parliament on Radio Four on 20 December 2020; the answer was that a vote could be held when Parliament returned in early January.
6. The regulations for the second lockdown were laid before Parliament at 4.10pm on Tuesday 3 November to be debated and voted on by MPs the following day and already advertised to come into effect at a minute past midnight on 5 November; peers also debated the SI on 4 November.
7. As the Parliament website (n.d.) explains: 'A money bill is a bill that in the opinion of the House of Commons Speaker is concerned only with national taxation, public money or loans. A bill that is certified as a money bill and which has been passed by the Commons will become law after one month, with or without the approval of the House of Lords, under the terms of the Parliament Acts.'
8. The figures used were themselves the subject of heated debate but the general message was clear: NHS funding is both necessary and politically popular.
9. The UK's most senior Finance Minister and one of the top roles in government.
10. For details of the various schemes, see House of Commons Library (2020a, 2020b).

Acknowledgements

The author would like to thank Charlie Fox for research assistance. She is grateful to Derek McDougall, William Wallace and David Yates as well as three anonymous reviewers for helpful comments on earlier drafts of the article.

Disclosure statement

Julie Smith is a member of the House of Lords. She writes in a personal capacity.

References

BBC News. (2020, September 11). *Nicola Sturgeon says Covid briefings "more important than ever"*. Retrieved November 1, 2020, from https://www.bbc.co.uk/news/uk-scotland-54115645

BBC Scotland News. (2020, October 27). *Covid in Scotland: The headlines*. Retrieved November 6, 2020, from https://www.bbc.co.uk/news/live/uk-scotland-54637236

Bercow, J. (2020, September 27). *The World this Weekend*.

Bevington, M. (2020). *What is an "Australian-style" deal?* UK in a Changing Europe. Retrieved December 14, 2020, from https://ukandeu.ac.uk/explainers/what-is-an-australian-style-deal/

Bowcott, O., Stewart, H., & Sparrow, A. (2020, September 20). Parliament surrendered role over Covid emergency laws, says Lady Hale. *The Guardian*.

Bradley, J., Gebrekidan, S., & McCann, A. (2020, December 17). Waste, negligence and cronyism - Inside Britain's pandemic spending. *New York Times*. Retrieved February 4, 2021 from: https://www.nytimes.com/interactive/2020/12/17/world/europe/britain-covid-contracts.html

Brewer, M., Cominetti, N., Henehan, K., McCurdy, C., Sehmi, R., & Slaughter, H. (2020). *Jobs, jobs, jobs – Evaluating the effects of the current economic crisis on the UK labour market*. Resolution Foundation. Retrieved October 28, 2020, from resolutionfoundation.org

Clatworthy, B., Waterfield, B., & Smyth, C. (2020, December 21). Europe shuts door on Britain over fears of mutant virus. *The Times*. Retrieved December 21, 2020, from https://www.thetimes.co.uk/edition/news/europe-shuts-door-on-britain-over-fears-of-mutant-virus-zzxghvsc8?utm_source=

newsletter&utm_campaign=newsletter_101&utm_medium=email&utm_content=101_11588420&CMP=TNLEmail_7172239_11588420_101

Colfer, B. (2020) 'Herd-immunity across intangible borders: Public policy responses to COVID-19 in Ireland and the UK', *European Policy Analysis*, *6*(2), 203–225. https://doi.org/10.1002/epa2.1096

Coronavirus Act 2020. (2020). https://www.legislation.gov.uk/ukpga/2020/7/pdfs/ukpga_20200007_en.pdf, last accessed 27 January 2021

Forsyth, L. (2020a, September 18). *HL Hansard*. 805, col. 1558-9.

Forsyth, L. (2020b, September 25). *HL Hansard*. 805, col. 2009–2010.

Hancock, M. (2020, March 23). *HC Hansard*. 674.

HM Treasury. (2020, November). *Spending Review 2020* (Presented to Parliament by the Chancellor of the Exchequer, CP 330).

Hope, C., & Dixon, H. (2020, May 1). The story behind "stay home, protect the NHS, save lives" – The slogan that was "too successful". *The Telegraph*. Retrieved October 28, 2020, from https://www.telegraph.co.uk/politics/2020/05/01/story-behind-stay-home-protect-nhs-save-lives/

House of Commons Library. (2020a, December 17). *Coronavirus business support schemes: Statistics briefing paper number CBP 8938*. Georgina Hutton and Matthew Keep. Retrieved December 20, 2020, from www.parliament.uk/commons-library/

House of Commons Library. (2020b, December 18). *Coronavirus: Support for businesses briefing paper number 8847*. Steve Browning. Retrieved December 20, 2020, from www.parliament.uk/commons-library/

House of Commons Public Administration and Constitutional Affairs Committee. (2020, September 10). *Parliamentary scrutiny of the government's handling of Covid-19* (Fourth Report of Session 2019-21 HC277) Oral Evidence

House of Lords Economic Affairs Committee. (2020). *Employment and COVID-19: Time for a new deal* (3rd Report of Session 2019-2021 HL Paper 188).

Johnson, B. (2020, October 31). Press conference. *BBC News*.

Kuenssberg, L. (2020, October 31). Coronavirus: Boris Johnson launches the nuclear option he swore to avoid. *BBC News*. Retrieved November 1, 2020, from https://www.bbc.co.uk/news/uk-politics-54766061

Morris, C. (2020). Brexit trade deal: What do WTO rules or an Australia-style relationship mean? *BBC News*. Retrieved December 14, 2020, from https://www.bbc.co.uk-45112872

Murray, P., & Matera, M. (2020). *"Australia-style": A model for relations with Europe?* UK in a Changing Europe. Retrieved December 14, 2020, from https://ukandeu.ac.uk/australia-style-a-model-for-relations-with-europe/

National Audit Office. (2020, November 26). *Investigation into government procurement during the COVID-19 pandemic* (HC959 Session 2019-2021).

NHS Providers. (2020, September). *Restoring services*. NHS Activity Tracker. www.nhsproviders.org/restoring-services-nhs-activity-tracker

NI Direct. (2020). *Coronavirus (COVID-19) regulations guidance: What the restrictions mean for you*. Retrieved November 1, 2020, from https://www.nidirect.gov.uk/articles/coronavirus-covid-19-regulations-guidance-what-restrictions-mean-you

Office for Budget Responsibility. (2020, November). *Economic and fiscal outlook* (CP 318).

Parliament website. (n.d.). *Money bills*. Retrieved November 6, 2020, from https://www.parliament.uk/site-information/glossary/money-bills/

Smith, J. (forthcoming 2021). And another thing: Parliament post Brexit. In B. Jones, P. Norton, & I. Hertner (Eds.), *Politics UK* (10th ed., forthcoming). Routledge.

Sumption, J. (2020, October 27). *Government by decree: Covid-19 and the constitution*. Cambridge Freshfields Annual Law Lecture. Retrieved November 1, 2020, from https://resources.law.cam.ac.uk/privatelaw/Freshfields_Lecture_2020_Government_by_Decree.pdf

Sunak, R. (2020, November 25). *Spending review 2020, statement by the Chancellor of the Exchequer*. House of Commons.

Swinford, S. (2020, November 6). Rishi Sunak's coronavirus support package "wasteful", says economist. *The Times*.

COVID-19 in Nigeria

Noo Saro-Wiwa

ABSTRACT
Drawing on the reactions of local experts in public health and health finance, this article traces the course of the pandemic in Nigeria, and discusses the measures taken to contain it, public compliance or non-compliance with those measures, and the inadequacy and under-funding of infection prevention methods. The article also assesses the pandemic situation in Port Harcourt and the thriving black market for food and other items on the Okike waterfront. The author asks whether the pandemic might be an opportunity to reorganise the Nigerian health care system, but is not optimistic.

Introduction

Watching the corona virus spread from China to Europe and then to Nigeria was like watching a tsunami develop. What starts as a curious ebbing of the waters becomes a wave on the horizon that draws closer while onlookers observe with curious detachment.

When news of the COVID-19 first made news headlines it was a problem in China only. Even as China imposed lockdown on the city of Wuhan where the virus originated, the world accepted it as a stringent action peculiar to the Communist Party.

'Our initial feeling was because there's a lot of trade between Nigeria and China,' says 'Temi', an Abuja-based public health expert with an international NGO (she does not want her real name used). 'We hadn't started seeing cases as they had in Europe and in the US. The initial thinking was, "Could there be something in our genetic makeup that was making us less susceptible to the disease?" Because for some reason we're not seeing cases and people are not dropping dead. And a lack of testing was not necessarily the reason why we're not seeing cases.'

Around late February, a fresh-faced 26-year-old woman walked into the government offices in Abuja to listen in to a COVID-19 strategy meeting.

'I had planned to travel in March,' says Asma'u Abiola, an associate in sustainable health financing. 'COVID-19 hadn't really hit. We didn't know what it was. So everyone thought, 'Just go ahead and do your thing, take time off.' But then things changed very quickly. The day I was supposed to leave I found out about this COVID-19. I have a close link to one of the people working on it, so I thought: before I hop on a flight to go anywhere, let me just find out more. Let's hear what people are saying, and how far along they are planning.

'I walk in. The governor of Kaduna state had gathered a small group of people. His chief of staff was there, and a senior person from Ekiti state. A couple of other states had sent their commissioners. And there were all these technical people. The World Bank sent two senior economists. So I'm thinking, "okay, this is really happening. This is serious".'

High-level casualties

Around the same time, a high number of high-level politicians were getting infected. Some people in that room had had very close contact with those people who we found out a week after that meeting were infected. So all of us were a bit scared. You'd literally [switch] on the TV and see someone who knows someone who you know was sitting with someone who has now been infected. You then feel that you now need to isolate. So it was very strange times at the end of March, beginning of April.'

Later that month, President Buhari's Chief of Staff, Abba Kyari, succumbed to the coronavirus. A highly influential member of the government 'Cabal', Kyari had been the president's gatekeeper. Anyone wanting an audience with the president had to go through him first. His death rocked political circles – and preceded a wave of big-name fatalities at the hands of COVID-19.

On June 25, the former governor of Oyo State, Abiola Ajimobi, passed away, followed by Wahab Adegbenro. State health officials panicked. As the Commissioner for Health in Ondo State, Adegbenro had led the task force against COVID-19. It is thought he may have contracted the virus from patients he had attended to in his private hospital.

The list of eminent COVID-19 sufferers grew longer. Several public officials tested positive for the virus but recovered, including the Governor of Ondo State Rotimi Akeredolu, Commissioner for Information Delta State Charles Aniagwu, and the governors of several states, including Abia, Bauchi, Oyo, Ekiti and Kaduna (*The Africa Report*, 17 July 2020).

Although the corona tsunami wave was now lapping on Nigeria's shores, the perception was that 'maybe it's only the politicians that it kills,' Temi says. The media was only reporting afflictions among Big Men, with their unfeasibly high salaries and luxury homes. 'Crony-virus' did not apply to low-income Nigerians.

Nigerian elites were flying into Lagos and Abuja from Europe and the US, trying to escape the pandemic, unaware that they were actually bringing it to Nigeria.

'Given what we were seeing in the news, and how it was bringing down Italy and starting to spread to France and Spain, we were surprised that our airports were still open,' Temi said. 'There was anger and confusion among us in the public health space as to why Nigeria was delaying its response.'

The political elite, not known for spreading the wealth, were helping to spread COVID-19. They gave generously to immigration officials, spouses, children, friends, civil servants, house servants, chauffeurs and waitresses. These low-income workers took the virus back to their 'Face-me-I-face-you' apartments, where crowded living conditions accelerated community transmission. Lagos, the nation's commercial capital, was the epicentre.

Its commercial links with northern cities like Kano put health officials in the northern region on alert. Soon enough, there was a jump in the number of unexplained burials in Kano, Jigawa, Sokoto and Yobe states. 'We all just flipped,' Temi says. Islamic culture was particularly COVID-19 friendly because of shoulder-to-shoulder group prayers in mosques, and not-so-flexible social customs. 'It's already difficult getting them to do anything related to formal health care. We started to see many northern states having a COVID-19 problem. The Muslim custom of burying bodies within 24-hours of death made it harder to ascertain whether COVID-19 was involved. A lot of these people were elderly and had co-morbidities. These were all signs of possible cases of COVID-19.'

To confuse matters further, state governments were not reporting their COVID-19 data. They feared accusations of pandemic mismanagement. 'We went through another two-month phase of these unreported deaths,' Temi said. 'They were coming up in the media but not showing up in the data.'

She says the federal government led an investigation into unreported deaths in Kano and concluded that up to 50% of the 1,000-plus unreported deaths may have been due to COVID-19. 'But the numbers were never adjusted to reflect that fact.'

Abiola, meanwhile, was enlisted to help the federal states strengthen the COVID-19 response. Her job entailed linking IPC (infection prevention and control) between the pillars of risk communications, case management, and testing and surveillance. She says it was very difficult initially to get other development planners on the table and strategise because the general belief was that they should focus less on prevention and more on testing, surveillance and case management.

'It would have been really cost-effective for us to invest more in infection prevention and control – hand-washing stations, sanitisers, triage stations, asking about travel history ... it's really simple stuff. And that's what's so frustrating. But, for whatever reason, it was not prioritised at the time. We don't invest in prevention as much. Our primary health care system is supposed to be preventative, but it's also the level of care that is least funded. The bulk of our budget goes towards overheads ... things like salaries.'

Financially, the pandemic battle couldn't have happened at a worse time. Parts of the global economy were at a near-standstill and oil prices had tumbled. 'We were thinking not just about the public health response, but also how we balance that with the economic response,' Abiola says. 'The whole 2020 budget no longer applies because all of the estimates have changed. We were projecting based on a price of US$55 per barrel. At this point, we were at a price of less than US$30. So a lot had changed very, very quickly. It was a mess.'

Talking to Abiola and Temi brought home to me the intellectual gulf between Nigerian health experts and the country's ineffectual politicians. It is a dichotomy that's played out in countries such as the United States where President Donald Trump clashed with infectious disease expert, Anthony Fauci.

'Sometimes the perception of the average Nigerian is that the authorities have no idea what they're doing,' Abiola says. 'But Dr Tochi Okwor [coordinator of IPC at the Nigeria Centre for Disease Control (NCDC)] is phenomenal. I don't know how she's not completely fatigued or bored of this whole thing, but she just keeps going at it. She is very, very technically sound, and I feel like if we as a country prioritised IPC a little bit more it would have been more effective in how things turned out, especially in the more populated states like Lagos.'

Port Harcourt

From the epicentre in the southwest region, COVID-19 spread rapidly to all geopolitical areas of Nigeria. Rivers State is the one of the world's most densely populated. There, the leadership's reaction to the pandemic mirrored the confusion and contradictions seen around the world.

The lockdown imposed on the southern city of Port Harcourt, my hometown, was sudden and severe. It was announced on a Sunday. Citizens were given until Tuesday – two days – to leave their jobs, hunker down at home and figure out alternative sources of income. Soldiers flogged people who were caught walking in the streets. The state governor cruised around town with an armed entourage and personally arrested individuals, says journalist Isaac Harry on Chicoco FM radio (Chicoco FM, 16 September 2020). They were sent to a 'quarantine centre' – a repurposed football stadium, to be exact – where distressed hoards were 'forced to huddle together under the sun for hours'.

Hard line and neglect

Having imposed movement restrictions in and out of Rivers State, government security agents detained 22 employees of the oil company ExxonMobil after they were caught entering the state from neighbouring Akwa Ibom (*Business Traffic*, 19 April 2020).

On Bonny island, the food supply chain was broken but the authorities had not provided any relief assistance. The army and police cracked down violently on people who flouted the lockdown curfew. Food prices soared and so did hunger. Hospitals were overwhelmed and began refusing to accept patients for fear of contamination. For a fortnight, the people of Bonny lived in fear. 'Buying and selling was done in the secret,' one resident told Chicoco FM radio (Chicoco FM, 1 August 2020).

So too were burial ceremonies. In early June, the state government introduced a law requiring that all public burials or movement of corpses out of the state be approved by the state governor. No more than 50 people could attend funerals. In response, people began burying their dead in secret. When the state governor's permanent secretary, Sunny Okere, allegedly attended a secret funeral service he was fired from his post.

But although the government took a hard line in some areas, it was neglectful in others. The proactive zeal with which it administered lockdown beatings and detentions seemingly disappeared over the more delicate and strategic matters of genuine infection prevention.

Over a busy road in the city centre, a billboard displays infection prevention advice. The wording is starchy and unidiomatic: *('Endeavour to practice good respiratory hygiene'); 'When sneezing or coughing, cover your mouth and nose with a tissue ... Then dispose off [sic] the used tissue safely, immediately.'* Why not communicate in Pidgin English, the true lingua franca? Surely it would connect better with a wider audience?

The advice on display also assumes Global North availability of urban space and medical resources: 'If you develop shortness of breath and other symptoms 'call doctor and seek care immediately' ... This, in a country where primary health care receives the least funding. 'Maintain at least one and a half metres (5 feet) distance.' Yes, but Port Harcourt's sidewalks are narrow and flanked by ditches.

People are told to refrain from giving handshakes and to greet others with 'a wave, nod or a bow instead.' Yet the authorities flouted all their own social distancing protocols when attempting to alleviate the food shortages created by the lockdown. Vehicles belonging to the government, private charities and church organisations cruised the streets, flinging food rations (tubers of yams and packets of Indomie instant noodles – known as 'palliatives') to hungry crowds. Jostling for position, people pleaded for their portion ('Give me!' ... 'Drop here!' ... 'My pikin, I never get, o!'). Men snatched packets out of young boys' hands. The scuffling and spittle-flecked arguments could only have aided viral transmission.

Food ration hand-outs only went so far. And so in the absence of proper government, welfare the informal sector – so crucial to Nigeria's economy – resumed its vital stop-gap role even if it was now illegal. After Port Harcourt's main market was closed, a thriving 'black market' soon sprang up – and in the most unlikely part of town.

Okrika waterfront lies at the southern end of Port Harcourt. Here, the river slows and divides into creeks that meander around islands. On the approach to the creekside neighbourhood, the tarred road peters out. Housing developers never built up this part of town as it is too prone to flooding. The area attracted poorer residents who built shanty homes along the swampy waterfront. During rainy season, the water levels rise and combine with the poor sanitation to make Okrika a no-go area. Rightly or wrongly, the neighbourhood has a reputation for crime, and most city dwellers – police included – generally give it a wide berth.

Yet at 2:00 a.m. one day, Tammy, an Okrika resident and journalist, woke up to see a procession of people passing by her house. 'Buckets and boxes and trays and bundles streamed past my window,' she said on Chicoco FM radio (Chicoco FM, 15 June 2020). When she asked her neighbour what was going on, the neighbour informed her that a new market had sprung up 'in the toilet, o!'

It turned out that Okrika's residents, many of whom are petty traders, had obtained permission from their local chairman to set up a pop-up market where they could sell their perishable stocks in contravention of the lockdown rules. Under the supervision of community youths, the market operated covertly in the early hours of the mornings.

The once-quiet road leading into Okrika waterfront was now filled with traders and buyers from neighbouring communities and beyond. Such was the desperation to obtain essentials that even the wealthy were sneaking over. Okrika's residents chortled at the sight of Lexus 350s, Range Rovers and Toyota Venzas rolling into their swamp ('They have forgotten their disdain!').

Despite their amusement, however, they could not ignore the glaring fact that nobody – buyers, sellers, rich or poor – appeared to give a damn about COVID-19. 'Money and goods change hands here,' Tammy and her colleagues remarked ... 'and so, no doubt, do germs.'

Ignorance or dismissal of infection risk was also a problem among Port Harcourt's law-enforcement who seemed to misunderstand the whys and wherefores of pandemic control and simply took advantage of the situation. This was illustrated in their treatment of Tammy's neighbour, a lady who had previously sold second-hand clothes but switched to selling corn (bought from Okrika's pop-up market) after losing all her customers during lockdown.

One day, as she stood on the roadside waiting for a taxi home, a truck pulled up. Inside it were shabbily attired Government Task Force men, none of whom wore masks or observed social distancing protocols. They jumped out and tried to confiscate the corn seller's produce. In the ensuing tussle she was tasered and slumped to the ground unconscious. When she came round minutes later, she discovered that her corn – and the soldiers – were gone.

Leadership was also lacking in the religious sphere. The COVID-19 billboard's advice to 'Stop Spreading Fake News on Social Media' applied to church pastors too. Some of them were doing their best to undermine the NCDC's prevention advice.

On Chicoco FM (28 August 2020), journalist Faithia Blaze describes attending church towards the end of April for the first time since lockdown. Christ Embassy Church on Aggrey Road, not far from my father's former office. An usher stood by the door, pouring sanitiser onto congregants' hands as they entered. When a lady asked him why he was doing this, the usher responded that he was following orders. He made no mention of the sanitary benefits.

On entering the church, Faithia discovered that she was the only congregant wearing a mask. It turns out that the pastor, a man in sharp black suit and matching shoes, mocked the idea of face covering. He likened the sight of a masked congregation to a 'Garden of zombies.' He continued: 'I want to tell you what the word of God says about masks.' On a screen he displayed Second Corinthians Chapter 4, Verse 2, and gave the audience his interpretation of it: '*But I renounce the hidden things of dishonesty, not working in craftiness*. We refuse to wear masks and play games. We are children of God. We will not wear masks. This virus will not be our portion if we know who we are!' The congregation hollered in affirmation.

Worshippers turned to Faithia and eyed her mask disapprovingly. In their opinion, it showed a lack of faith in God's protection. After the service, one female congregant told Faithia that her only reason for wearing a mask outdoors was to avoid 'embarrassment' from the police.

Non-compliance

The refusal to comply with COVID-19 measures seems to span different cultures, from Brazil to the United States and Nigeria. Ostensibly, the reasons differ (Nigerian Pentecostalism, Trumpist patriotism, etc.) but the defiance seems rooted in some instinct that unifies us all – perhaps a desperation to return to normal, or a belief that economic collapse represents a bigger existential threat than the virus.

Domestic flights into Port Harcourt resumed on July 11. That month, there were 1,088 confirmed COVID-19 cases and 38 deaths in Rivers State. By July 31, that number had risen to 1,791 and 52 respectively. Armageddon did not happen. A total of 600,000 Nigerians were tested – a small fraction of a population that's estimated at 170 million minimum.

'Nationally, we're still under 60,000 cases,' Abiola says, 'but that's probably [multiplied] by god-knows what.'

Temi says that by October 2020 testing had dropped significantly. 'Because it did not decimate the population, we're seeing poor compliance with all of the risk measures, even amongst the educated middle classes.'

'People, are just over it,' Abiola adds. 'People are bored of the topic. They are very fatigued.'

Temi recalls the time she reprimanded a local shopkeeper for not wearing a mask or providing hand sanitiser to his customers. He replied, 'Auntie, forget that one, jor! There is no COVID! Nigeria is just cooking up the numbers. If there is COVID, why aren't we seeing the people who are dying on TV? In Italy in America, they're showing us their hospital wards every day. In Nigeria they're not showing us any war. It's only when one politician dies that we hear that the politician has died!'

The complacency surrounding COVID-19, though frustrating, is understandable. 'There was a time when we were getting 10 deaths today, nine deaths, the next day, Temi says. 'Now it's like zero deaths in the last week. As a medical person my instinct is that if this thing was as severe as we expected it to be then our hospitals should be overwhelmed with cases by now. But still, we're not seeing our hospitals overflowing. A lot of people who probably gotten the infection by now, myself included, I don't know. And we've recovered fine, maybe a mild illness here or there. They're not seeing it really kill people. So there's this nonchalance in the general population.

'The other narrative I've heard from the community is that there are bigger issues to contend with. COVID-19 is the least of our problems. Poverty is killing us. Hunger is killing us. Malaria has been killing us since forever.'

Is such an argument wrong? I ask.

'I don't think it's wrong,' Temi tells me, 'but I don't think that one disease takes pre-eminence over another. Because our systems are generally weak and all human development indices are so low, we have a myriad of problems, and that was manifesting. Because COVID-19 is a pandemic, this is something that crosses borders. And we see that now it's affected more than 30 million people globally, with over 1 million deaths. It's a lot. It may seem small when you compare it to how many Nigerians or Africans have been dying from malaria and HIV and other diseases, but this is still a disease that killed over 1 million people in six months.

And it has changed the way we do everything. The way we do business, the way we travel. It's impacting the economy in ways that many of these other geographically localised diseases have not. While COVID-19 may not seem like a major problem [compared to] malaria or maternal deaths, and so on, it has crippled even the best health care systems in the world. We have seen the Italian hospitals overrun. It's just a different problem. That's how I see it.

COVID is a novel disease. We don't know how this thing is going to evolve with time. One of the conversations happening right now in the clinical setting is putting in place systems to understand the associated after-effects of COVID-19 infection, because there have been some reports of people who don't ever seem to really recover from it. Or at least we don't know how long it takes to fully recover.

And it is an expensive disease because of the hospitalisation costs. It has the potential to deplete the health care system as well. Research is needed to examine the potential damage the virus can wreak on other organs. We really need to understand what has reduced the severity among Africans because definitely it was reduced.' There are other theories about cross immunity from vaccines such as BCG for tuberculosis. The word on the street is that almost everybody self medicates due to the broken health care system. Drugs that should be prescription-only are freely available off-the-counter. 'For every little ailment, such as back pain, people are just popping pills. People have pumped themselves with cocktails of medicines that may have reduced the severity of COVID-19 ... who knows? Also, people have been using chloroquine. And despite the evidence from the West that chloroquine does not work, I have seen, based on the work that I do – and I'm not exaggerating – even teaching hospitals using chloroquine to manage COVID patients.'

Will this pandemic prove to be a turning point for Nigerian health care system? I ask. Temi sees it as an opportunity to reorganise our health care spaces, to build a functioning surveillance system and establish the right accountability measures.

'This should be our opportunity to strengthen the health care system so that we don't even have to continue dying from malaria and all these other diseases that have been plaguing us for years. A lot of people thought maybe this is the turning point. Now that all our politicians are stuck here, they can't go outside of the country to get treatment.'

However, Temi is not so optimistic: 'Because I've worked with government long enough now to see that it's all just talk. On paper, they're making all these declarations, but those of us who work inside the system … we know that they're doing *jack*. It's still about personal gain … who's making money off this pandemic. There's no real commitment. Everybody's just back to thinking, Thank God I made it. Thank God flights are now open. We can go back to flying to Houston and London, or wherever, to get health care. 'And they cut down health care while we were in a pandemic! Can you believe that? Where's the commitment to making things better for the average Nigerian?'

Abiola added 'Even if we then decided that we want to do better we don't have as much money as we used to. There were times when we literally could have done anything and everything for education, health and social security, but we didn't do it.' As a proportion of federal budget spending, Abiola says health spending peaked way back in 2012 at just 6%. 'So I don't see how we'll do it now that we're so much worse off financially.'

Conclusion: misplaced priorities

The slashing of crude oil revenues does not appear to have realigned the federal government's priorities. It appropriated N27 billion to renovate the National Assembly (*The Guardian*, 4 June 2020). Although the director-general for the budget office insisted that the allocated budget was slashed by 75%, it still means N7 billion has gone towards renovations at the expense of health. '*During* COVID,' Abiola exclaims. 'That tells you everything.'

Disclosure statement

No potential conflict of interest was reported by the author.

References

The Africa Report. (2020, July 17). Not even Nigeria's political elite can hide from coronavirus. (https://www.theafricareport.com/33910/not-even-nigerias-political-elite-can-hide-from-coronavirus/)

Business Traffic. (2020, April 19). Security agencies arrest, quarantine 22 Exxon workers in Rivers State. https://businesstraffic.com.ng/security-agencies-arrest-quarantine-22-exxon-workers-in-rivers-state/

Chicoco FM. (2020, August 1). Pandemic timeline. https://chicoco.fm/pandemic-timeline-july/

Chicoco FM. (2020, August 28). Small potatoes and the great unmasking. https://chicoco.fm/small-potatoes-and-the-great-unmasking/

Chicoco FM. (2020, June 15). Bad hood good market. https://chicoco.fm/bad-hood-good-market/

Chicoco FM. (2020, September 16). Chicoco crew: Covering corona. https://chicoco.fm/chicoco-crew-covering-corona/

The Guardian. Budget Office denies allocating N27 billion for National Assembly renovation. (2020, June 4). https://guardian.ng/news/budget-office-denies-allocating-n27-billion-for-national-assembly-renovation/

Malaysia, Myanmar and Singapore: common threads, divergences, and lessons learned in responding to the COVID-19 pandemic

Kyaw San Wai, Wai Yee Krystal Khine, Jane Mingjie Lim, Pearlyn Hui Min Neo, Rayner Kay Jin Tan and Suan Ee Ong

ABSTRACT

The COVID-19 pandemic has served as a prolonged global stress test in 2020. Southeast Asia is geographically and economically close to China, where COVID-19 first emerged. The region is home to diverse populations, densely packed cities, and a varied assortment of countries all across the development ladder. This article explores the multi-faceted COVID-19 responses of three countries in Southeast Asia – Malaysia, Myanmar and Singapore – countries who share a common history of British colonisation. This article explores the three countries' overall responses to the pandemic, highlighting shared challenges and divergences based on their respective experiences: Singapore as an advanced, highly urbanised city-state; Malaysia as an advanced developing country; and Myanmar as a lower-resourced developing country.

Introduction

The COVID-19 pandemic has served as a prolonged stress test on the globe in 2020. One of the most pressing acute public health crises in the past 100 years and amplified by globalisation, this pandemic has impacted almost every aspect of society. Growing major power rivalries in an increasingly multipolar world, the spread of populist and hyper-partisan politics and a zeitgeist coloured by climate change, rising inequality and social media have hampered effective global coordination. The concomitant infodemic has seen countries' responses prematurely praised or criticised, with numerous conspiracy theories and misinformation percolating and gaining traction as governments and societies grappled with evolving and dynamic new circumstances.

Southeast Asia is geographically and economically close to China, where COVID-19 first emerged. The region is home to diverse populations, densely-packed cities, and a varied assortment of countries all across the development ladder. This article will explore the multi-faceted COVID-19 responses of three countries in Southeast Asia – Malaysia, Myanmar and Singapore – countries who share a common history of British colonisation.[1] We discuss the common threads and the pertinent issues faced in these countries' responses to COVID-19.

COVID-19 in Malaysia, Myanmar, and Singapore: outbreak challenges and responses

Malaysia

Malaysia's first three COVID-19 cases were reported on 25 January 2020, all foreign nationals entering the country through Singapore. The first local case was identified on 4 February. That same month, a large-scale religious conference of over 16,000 attendees took place at Kuala Lumpur's Jamek Sri Petaling Mosque (Beech, 2020a). More than 600 cases were linked to the mosque cluster by the end of March, and almost half of Malaysia's total cases were attributed to the cluster by mid-May (Ananthalakshmi & Sipalan, 2020). Following the country's first two deaths, the government enacted a Movement Control Order (MCO) on 18 March that prohibited mass movements and gatherings, restricted travel into the country, and closed all non-essential services, including education institutions and other government and private establishments. On 27 March, an Enhanced MCO was enacted in areas reporting increased daily case numbers. By the end of April, cases had declined substantially and most economic sectors were reopened on 4 May with social distancing measures and a continued ban on mass gatherings and interstate travel under the new Conditional MCO. On 10 June, the government enacted the Recovery MCO, which resumed interstate travel and some religious gatherings. Mandatory mask-wearing in public places was introduced from 1 August following the emergence of new clusters. However, new clusters emerged across the states of Sabah, Selangor, Negeri Sembilan, Johor, Penang, and Kedah in September, leading to a resurgence of cases nationwide.

Overall, Malaysia responded fairly rapidly and cohesively to COVID-19. The National Security Council (NSC) mobilised the national response with technical guidance from the Ministry of Health (MOH). Five days after the first cases were reported, MOH published guidelines and established designated COVID-19 management hospitals nationwide. Some government hospitals, such as non-specialist hospitals, were converted into full or partial COVID-19 hospitals and hotels were converted into quarantine facilities (World Health Organization, 2020). Over the course of the outbreak, Malaysia increased its daily testing capacity and rolled out initiatives such as a contact tracing application,[2] drive-through screening services and Field Hybrid Intensive Care Units (ICU). Risk communication continues in the form of regular media briefings and digital and social media messaging. Additionally, the Malaysian government has worked to support its citizens and bolster the socioeconomic impacts of the pandemic via MYR305 billion (US$73.7 billion) worth of stimulus packages that include tax incentives, financial support for businesses and wage subsidies (KPMG, 2020).

Myanmar

Myanmar confirmed its first two COVID-19 cases on 23 March 2020, from visiting emigrants. The country had implemented airport screening since early January and had sent back an inbound flight on 31 January after one of the passengers developed symptoms. The first local transmission was reported on 27 March, with the outbreak mostly in Yangon. The country severed all international air travel on 31 March, and a 'Stay-at-Home Order' (SAHO) was imposed in affected townships in mid-April. The government adopted a 'Containment-at-source' strategy, mandating all confirmed cases to receive treatment in government health facilities, aggressively quarantined contacts and implemented localised lockdowns. In June, as the situation improved, SAHOs were eased. However, the return of over 150,000 migrant workers from Thailand and China (International Labour Organization, ILO, 2020), with some who circumvented COVID-19 checks, overwhelmed border checkpoints, further raising concerns about effective containment. Up till mid-August, the country had reported only 374 cases and six deaths. However, from mid-August, Myanmar started experiencing a much larger COVID-19 outbreak that began in Sittwe, the regional capital of strife-torn Rakhine State, which subsequently spread to other major cities. On 9 September, Yangon went back under SAHO, with other cities and towns soon following suit. International flights remain suspended until the end of 2020, and public schools, religious buildings and entertainment venues have mostly remained closed since March. Although different ordinances, including mandatory mask wearing and a ban on large public gatherings, have been imposed, enforcement has been patchy, especially in Yangon.

While COVID-19 test samples were sent initially to Thailand, the government has since expanded testing capacity. Currently, around 6000 polymerase chain reaction (PCR) tests are being performed daily, alongside over 15,000 using rapid antigen test kits. The containment-at-source approach that initially worked well imposed tremendous stress on the fragile health system during the second outbreak (Naing, 2020). Over 200,000 people were reportedly quarantined across housing projects, schools and military camps between mid-August and October, while asymptomatic patients volunteered or were drafted to assist health staff. The government only began exploring for private facilities to treat COVID-19 in October (Angel, 2020).

Myanmar established a number of inter-ministerial committees to coordinate the COVID-19 response, with the main 'National-level Central Committee on Prevention, Control and Treatment of Covid-19' headed by State Counsellor Aung San Suu Kyi. The Covid-19 Economic Relief Plan (CERP) was announced in late April, valued at around US$3 billion, under which regular cash transfers to households, loans to struggling businesses and wage provision to formal-sector workers were implemented. In late September, a longer-term Myanmar Economic Recovery and Reform Plan (MERRP) was announced (Tun, 2020).

Singapore

Singapore moved early and quickly to manage COVID-19. The government had paid keen attention to COVID-19's spread, watching developments in China, Japan, Hong Kong and South Korea that ultimately informed their pre-emptive measures. Temperature screenings for incoming flights from Wuhan were implemented on 3 January 2020 and from 20 January, travellers with respiratory symptoms and a 14-day travel history to China were isolated. Two days later, the government convened a Multi-Ministry Task Force comprising representatives from across the health, manpower, finance, trade and industry sectors to lead the national COVID-19 response. The next day, a tourist from Wuhan was confirmed as Singapore's first COVID-19 case. Seven days and nine additional confirmed cases later, on 30 January, the World Health Organization declared COVID-19 a Public Health Emergency of International Concern. By 7 February, the national Disease Outbreak Response System Condition (DORSCON) level was raised from Yellow to Orange after cases with untraceable origins surfaced. Singapore's borders remain closed to tourists and strict quarantine measures are in place for returning residents.

Domestically, a lockdown termed the 'Circuit Breaker' (CB) was implemented from 7 April to 1 June. Meanwhile, Singapore's Government Technology Agency launched digital tools to facilitate contact tracing and information dissemination. Plans to gradually reopen economic activity in three phases were announced. Civil society efforts, including grassroots initiatives focused on mask distribution and migrant worker assistance, helped create space and opportunities to address the psychosocial impact of COVID-19 on vulnerable communities. Since the pandemic began, the government has announced SG$100.5 billion (US$74 billion) worth of spending across five stimulus packages. At the time of writing, Singapore was in Phase 2 of its reopening; the taskforce had announced plans to transition to Phase 3 by the end of the year, citing economic and vaccine availability considerations (Awang, 2020). As of early December 2020, Singapore boasted only 80 active cases and 29 deaths out of 58,285 confirmed cases and the lowest COVID-19 case-fatality rate in the world – 0.05% compared to the global average of 4.34%. However, several blind spots precluded a seamless response to the pandemic, including a dip in surgical mask supplies in early 2020 leading to a price surge, mixed messaging around the need for and efficacy of mask-wearing, and widespread disease transmission in low-wage migrant worker dormitories (Yi et al., 2020).

Key issues and lessons

Pandemic preparedness and response

As a major hotspot for zoonoses (Bordier & Roger, 2013) and infectious diseases, the Southeast Asia region has been afflicted by notable disease such as SARS, H5N1 ('bird flu'), H1N1 ('swine flu'), Nipah virus, drug-resistant malaria, dengue fever, Zika, Chikungunya, Japanese encephalitis and MERS since 2000. With its first-hand experience of the SARS epidemic combined with its status as a major global transit hub, Singapore has invested significant resources in maintaining a pandemic preparation and response capacity (Lin, Lee & Lye, 2020) including serving as a regional technical and academic resource base, and in cultivating multilateral initiatives. Malaysia's travel and tourism links, heavy land border traffic with Thailand and Singapore, and its zoonotic disease challenges arising from its rich tropical biodiversity have also been underlying factors for investing in infectious disease surveillance and response. Myanmar's infectious disease burden – particularly tuberculosis, dengue and malaria – and its location within the Greater Mekong Subregion zoonotic hotspot led to domestic and international efforts to strengthen disease surveillance.

All three countries implemented airport screening in early January, with a special focus on flights arriving from China. Air travel with China was restricted and subsequently suspended by all three countries in late January and early February. Once community transmissions were detected in-country, the three quickly implemented population-wide lockdowns under varying guises and a strong emphasis on contact tracing, quarantines, cluster identification and targeted responses. All three countries also pursued a maximum containment approach where all confirmed COVID-19 cases were either hospitalised or mandated to be isolated. The public also proactively began wearing facemasks, long before health authorities had confirmed COVID-19's actual mode of transmission.

While these were critical factors in allowing the countries to prepare for COVID-19, their health systems nonetheless faced tremendous strain when widespread community transmission occurred, especially in Malaysia's Sabah state and Myanmar's Yangon region. Mirroring reports from COVID-19 hotspots around the world, stories emerged of health systems pushed to the brink. Reflecting their more advanced and better resourced medical systems, both Singapore and Malaysia have registered low case-fatality rates compared to Myanmar.

Singapore was in many ways extremely prepared to tackle COVID-19 thanks to a confluence of several factors: a firm-handed government that took a whole-of-government approach and swiftly, decisively implemented comprehensive movement control policies; the economic capacity to alleviate the impact of such policies; and experiences with SARS, which exposed key weaknesses in the country's surveillance and healthcare systems and led to a series of broad reforms in the healthcare system. These reforms included the establishment of a crisis management plan and the DORSCON system, which provides a colour-coded, tiered national response system that considers the nature of the disease threat, impact of the response on daily life, and advice to the public. Singapore has benefited from an increased health systems capacity to handle emerging infectious diseases, with more isolation facilities in public hospitals, a purpose-built national centre for infectious diseases, and improved training and availability of infectious disease physicians. Singapore had also learnt from SARS the importance of effective public education and communication during a pandemic (Lin et al., 2020).

Likewise, Malaysia's ability to respond to COVID-19 was in no small part bolstered by the building blocks of government investment in the health system over the past decade. Between 2010 and 2018, the Malaysian government allocated MYR193.6 billion (US$46.7 billion) to the provision of healthcare services (Ministry of Finance Malaysia, 2019). In 2019, the Pakatan Harapan (PH) government allocated the Ministry of Health MYR28.7 billion (US$6.9 billion), which was increased to MYR31 billion (US$7.5 billion) in 2020. Although this investment was substantial and amounted to 2% of GDP, this budget was criticised for failing to meet the ruling coalition's manifesto promise of investing 4% of GDP into health (Khor, 2019); not addressing fundamental healthcare financing issues like the development of a universal national health insurance scheme; and focusing on strengthening secondary care rather than primary care (Durgahyeni, 2019). Recently, the government once again came under fire for announcing its Budget 2021 that allocated only RM31.9 billion to the Ministry of Health in the midst of a global pandemic – a mere 4.3% increase from its RM30.6 billion allocation in the 2020 budget. Concerningly, the 2021 budget further reduces the Ministry of Health's medical budget by 20.5% from 2020, including cuts across pharmacy and supplies (e.g. drugs, personal protective equipment, or PPE), public health, and non-communicable disease areas (e.g. kidney disease, cancer care, psychiatry and mental health) (Ravindran, 2020). It remains unclear what the new budget's implications for pandemic response will be as Malaysia continues to face high daily case counts into the new year.

In Myanmar, despite significant increase in public financing over recent years, its health system remains one of the weakest in Southeast Asia. Since reforms began in 2011, government health spending climbed from MMK85 billion (US$98 million) to MMK1.17 trillion (US$820 million, around US$15 per person) for FY2019-2020, representing 3.3% of the government budget and 0.9% of GDP. Around 74% of total health spending derives from out-of-pocket payments at the point of care, the highest in Southeast Asia. The country was set to introduce a Basic-Essential Package of Health Services (B-EPHS) for Universal Health Coverage in 2021 under the latest National Health Plan, but the effect of COVID-19 on health financing and further policy prioritisation remains to be seen. While the country has experience responding to emerging and re-emerging infectious diseases and its health system is being strengthened using bilateral and multilateral donor support (e.g., the Global Fund to Fight AIDS, Tuberculosis and Malaria), its pandemic preparedness capacity is relatively limited compared to its regional neighbours. The country's response has been buttressed by donations from regional countries, international partners and its private sector. Civil society has also played a key role in filling gaps in essential services, with community ambulances and welfare organisations mainly responsible for transporting patients and manning of quarantine facilities. However, as cases surged after mid-August, much of the health infrastructure came close to being overwhelmed and contact tracing appeared to have been suspended after the first few thousand cases.

COVID elections

All three countries held elections in 2020. Singapore and Myanmar held general elections in July and November 2020 respectively; meanwhile, Malaysia held state elections in September, but in a strange twist was the only country among the three to see a change in government. Although not the deciding factor of election outcomes, COVID-19 brought the shifting political sands of all three countries into greater focus.

Malaysia saw the collapse of its first-ever non-Barisan Nasional (National Front, or BN) coalition government amid internal power struggles and shock political moves. Defections of several lawmakers for the then ruling PH coalition and the resignation of Prime Minister Mahathir Mohamad precipitated in the dissolution of parliament, and the appointment of Muhyiddin Yassin as Prime Minister by the King on 29 February. By 17 May, a new coalition, Perikatan Nasional – in alliance with UMNO/BN – had taken over the reins of government. Recently, the new government came under fire for its pandemic management. After a sustained period of near zero locally transmitted cases, districts across Malaysia saw a surge in cases following a snap state election in the vast East Malaysian state of Sabah. High volumes of movement to and within Sabah took place during the campaign period leading up to election day on 26 September 2020, with interstate travel allowed and mandatory in-person voting giving rise to an influx of out-of-state Sabahans returning to vote. Over a million voters turned out to vote physically at designated polling stations state-wide. While reported voter compliance to safe voting measures was high, physical rallies of unlimited attendees in open spaces and up to 250 individuals in enclosed spaces were allowed, increasing transmission risk during the pre-election campaigning period (Povera & Chan, 2020; *Malay Mail*, 2020a). Interstate voters and travellers coming to Sabah from other parts of Malaysia (e.g., politicians, campaign workers) did not have to undergo 14-day quarantine upon return to their states of residence (Bunyan, 2020). Post-election increases in COVID-19 case counts have since been reported nationwide, with a record high of 2,188 new cases on 24 November 2020 (Ministry of Health, Malaysia, 2020). On 9 November, a nationwide Conditional MCO was reinstated, with the exception of three low-transmission states and an Enhanced MCO was extended across states reporting new emergent clusters. In light of the severe ramifications of the Sabah state election on national COVID-19 case counts, the Malaysian King declared a state of emergency to postpone a by-election for Sabah's Batu Sapi parliamentary constituency, initially slated for 5 December (V Tan, 2020).

Meanwhile, in Myanmar, the incumbent National League for Democracy (NLD) led by State Counsellor Aung San Suu Kyi managed to expand its majority in parliament, securing 77.46% of all elected seats in the union and state/region levels with a 71% turnout. This was in contradiction to tealeaf reading by both domestic and external analysts. Citing security concerns, the Union Election Commission (UEC) cancelled voting in certain ethnic minority areas that affected 1.5 million out of 38 million eligible voters affected. As the elections were held while Myanmar was in the midst of its second outbreak, there were concerns that the polls could lead to more cases. However, NLD party leaders stated that the elections were of equal importance to the pandemic and supporters raised the spectre of an unelected caretaker government. The UEC implemented advance voting for those over the age of 60 and opened extra polling stations. The government also reported purchasing over 35 million N95 masks and millions of units of PPE for use in the election (Myanmar News Agency, 2020). Electioneering saw large crowds outside of Yangon, where the SAHO barred gatherings. However, huge crowds celebrating the NLD's landslide victory broke many COVID ordinances and have been blamed for an increase in cases since mid-November.

Compared to many countries, Myanmar's civilian government operates in a tighter space due to the country's complicated relationship with the military that maintains a powerful and autonomous praetorian role in domestic politics. This has translated into an unwillingness to deploy the security sector to enforce SAHOs. Furthermore, the military-linked former ruling party and its allies tried to push for the convening of the military-dominated National Defence and Security Council (Moe, 2020). This prompted the government to adopt a number of workarounds, relying instead on the General Administration Department (GAD), which had only been transferred to civilian control at the end of 2018, to oversee SAHOs. It also formed a Control and Emergency Response Committee headed by the military-nominated First Vice President and included the three ministries controlled by the Tatmadaw and military officials, alongside relevant civilian ministries, to coordinate safety and security-related issues.

Singapore held its General Election on 10 July 2020. Prime Minister Lee Hsien Loong justified the decision to call fresh polls mid-pandemic to "give the new government a fresh five-year mandate" (Beech, 2020b). The election was shaped by the election in two major ways: first, the election's main issues were shaped by the pandemic, namely criticism over the government's handling of the pandemic and concerns over a potential post-pandemic economic recession. Second, the pandemic changed the way campaigning and voting took place. Politicians reoriented their campaigns away from physical rallies, which were disallowed, and towards television, the internet, Zoom, banners, socially distanced walkabouts, and perambulating vehicles that proclaimed party manifestos and election promises from loudspeakers. On polling day, safe management measures for voters, like physical distancing, temperature taking and hand hygiene, were enforced. Special voting time slots were allocated to vulnerable populations, like the elderly. These measures led to reduced voting efficiency and long queues at polling stations – an unusual experience for Singaporean voters who are accustomed to highly efficient voting procedures. However, there was no recorded spike in COVID-19 cases in the community in the immediate post-election period, suggesting the effectiveness of election safety measures. Ultimately, the incumbent PAP won 83 out of 93 seats but received 61.24% of the popular vote, its lowest showing in a decade.

Governance

Each of the countries took unique approaches to governance during the pandemic. Although all three chose to communicate risk in a reassuring and calm way, lean into the use of media for information sharing and approach vaccine access with a broadly open strategy, their standard operating procedure and safe distancing enforcement efforts, levels of trust in government and institutions and use of technologies for contact tracing varied.

The Malaysian government employed a risk communication approach grounded in constancy and reassurance, with clear figureheads in the fight against COVID-19. Health Director-General Noor Hisham Abdullah has become the public face of the pandemic, becoming a familiar, trusted, apolitical leader of health system frontliners and reliable conveyor of statistics and evolving scientific evidence. Although Prime Minister Muhyiddin Yassin has stepped up to deliver routine speeches during the pandemic, his use of colloquial and often paternalistic language, such as referring to himself as *'abah'* ('father'), has been criticised as a theatrical attempt to endear himself to a population that did not vote his government into power. Social media was somewhat leaned into, with Twitter and Telegram emerging as main information dissemination nodes. Meanwhile, the government is working to develop better understandings of the relationship between quality and effectiveness of communication on public behaviour, the impacts of information fatigue and misinformation, how to build better public trust in institutions, and how to shift narratives away from fear and towards optimism and progress (*Malay Mail*, 2020b).

Authorities also took a progressive and incremental approach to enforcing safe distancing measures (Tang, 2020). Examples included instituting roadblocks across the country and mobilising military forces to ensure enforcement and adherence to prohibitions around movement of persons during lockdown. These actions were further reinforced with fines and potential prison sentences for flouting COVID-19 standard operating procedures, including masking and quarantine orders. However, public outcry of double standards surfaced when authorities were found to have exercised leniency on politicians who had disregarded such procedures (Jaipragas, 2020). The MySejahtera contact tracing mobile app was developed to facilitate nationwide contact tracing efforts. However, as of August 2020, there has been only 60% uptake at population level. Authorities considered mandating the use of the app but at time of writing, this has not yet been enforced. On the vaccine front, the government has signed agreements with pharmaceutical giant Pfizer for 12.8 million vaccine doses and with COVAX, an initiative supporting global equitable access to vaccines, for another 3 million. The government aims to vaccinate 30% of the population by the end of 2021 (Channel News Asia, 2020). Distribution will be free, with priority given to high-risk groups, including healthcare professionals and people living with multiple illnesses. However, challenges remain, including cold chain and logistics and politically sensitive decisions around whether or not to vaccinate certain high-risk groups, like prisoners and detainees.

Meanwhile, the Myanmar government leaned heavily into social media to effectively convey COVID-19 updates and information to the public. The Ministry of Health and Sports' (MOHS) official Facebook page following grew from 700,000 in December 2019 to 6 million by December 2020. The government's COVID-19 message group on the Viber platform has 1.9 million subscribers, allowing for highly effective information sharing in a country with a mobile penetration rate of over 95%. In northern Rakhine, a much-criticised internet ban due to spiralling conflict was perceived as a major hurdle by activists. However, the government reported conducting information campaigns including utilising handheld speakers and radio-broadcasts, including in Bengali for Rohingya communities (Ministry of Health and Sports, Myanmar, 2020). MOHS also disseminated posters in various ethnic languages across the country, especially for internally displaced persons' camps across different states. While the government developed the Saw Saw Shar mobile contact tracing app, it has been downloaded only over 100,000 times, with very little use. The government has adopted a reassuring tone in its communications, partly influenced by domestic political sensitivities and tenuous civil-military relations. Although State Counsellor Aung San Suu Kyi has been the most visible public face of the national response, there remains no dedicated COVID-19 spokesperson. The head of Yangon's main COVID-19 facility began giving daily press briefings in late September with a more frank risk assessment, but the initiative lost steam by mid-October (Htwe, 2020). The government and the general public also took to emphasising the daily positivity rate above all other metrics to gauge the control of the outbreak.

Enforcement of safe distancing remains a key obstacle, rooted in a lack of capacity, bureaucracy, new ordinances issued on very short notice, and the country's political culture. Endemic corruption has caused the public to conflate enforcement with extortion and respond poorly to fines. Also, while Yangon's regional government initially introduced a ban on travel between different townships, enforcement soon petered out. Myanmar has taken an open approach to access to a COVID-19 vaccine: it has signed up to COVAX and the World Bank has pledged support to assist with loans for vaccine purchases and cold chain upgrades. Myanmar's balancing relations between China and India are also reflected in it being declared or hinted as a prioritised candidate to receive domestically-developed vaccines from both countries (CGTN, 2020; Chaudhury, 2020). Overall, despite the steep learning curve and various shortcomings, the pandemic has been a 'baptism by fire' for the NLD government. Given Aung San Suu Kyi's continued and immense popularity, the Myanmar public has generally been supportive of the government's handling of the pandemic and relatively forgiving of shortfalls.

In contrast, Singapore grounded its pandemic risk communication in 'defensive pessimism', as practised during SARS in 2003 (Wong, 2020). This meant that COVID-19 risks were framed as serious, not to be underestimated and likely to persist, with emphasis on government responsibility to prepare for challenges and uncertainty ahead. The Multi-Ministry Taskforce took the lead on regularly updating the public on daily statistics and new scientific developments, including emerging evidence around disease transmission and vaccine developments. They became especially visible and subject to public scrutiny and criticism following Singapore's large-scale migrant worker dormitory outbreak, which is detailed later in this paper. Complementarily, Prime Minister Lee Hsien Loong's nationwide addresses would focus more on the announcement of major policies and/or 'checking in' with the public to reassure them of ongoing efforts to cushion them from the adverse impacts of the pandemic, including stimulus packages and job support schemes. Conscious efforts were made to deliver news of key announcements in a culturally competent manner: for example, the Prime Minister's nationally televised announcement of a nationwide circuit breaker was made in three languages – English, Malay, and Mandarin Chinese. Singapore authorities also utilised both conventional media and new media to communicate COVID-19 information to the public, including digital tools like WhatsApp and Telegram. All these efforts took place against the backdrop of relatively high population-level levels of trust in government and institutions (Lim et al., 2020).

Perhaps unsurprisingly, the Singapore government established stringent, clear guidelines for safe distancing early in the pandemic, including physical distancing and mask-wearing once the scientific evidence strongly suggested their role in preventing COVID-19 transmission. These were further reinforced by severe punishments for flouting of safe distancing guidelines, including work pass revocation and/or deportations of foreign nationals, fines or imprisonment for locals, and fines and closure orders for food and beverage and other retail outlets. A form of social policing has also been enacted: members of the community termed 'safe distancing ambassadors' rove around public spaces to ensure that people stay one metre apart and wear masks at all times. Like neighbouring Malaysia, Singapore has a contact tracing app: TraceTogether. Also, like Malaysia, despite efforts to encourage app downloads and use, uptake in the population remains low – public health experts and government officials alike agree that this low uptake is a key barrier to Singapore advancing to its third phase of economic reopening (Chong & Begum, 2020). However, unlike Malaysia and more like Myanmar, Singapore has chosen to take an open approach to accessing COVID-19 vaccines (A. Tan, 2020; Teo, 2020). Government officials have explicitly stated that there is 'no need' to rely on just one vaccine given there are multiple vaccines in the race, electing instead to focus on safety and efficacy. At time of writing, American biotechnology company Moderna is seeking approval for use of its vaccine in Singapore, with the aim of being approved by the end of December 2020. Singapore is also part of COVAX, but on the other side: it is part of a multilateral group of high-income nations called Friends of COVAX who are committed to supporting equitable COVID-19 vaccine access in low- and middle-income countries, including its immediate Southeast Asian neighbours.

Vulnerable populations

Another shared challenge of the three countries is how to manage and control COVID-19 is vulnerable populations, including labour migrants, internal migrants, refugees, internally displaced persons and detainees. As early as May 2020, clusters had been identified at immigration depots, detention centres, and construction sites staffed by migrant workers in Peninsular Malaysia. Numbers have remained worrying ever since. In October 2020, new cases in Sabah – already reeling from the post-election spike in cases – were traced to a detention centre that housed illegal migrant workers from Indonesia and the Philippines (*The Straits Times*, 2020a). November saw high levels of COVID-19 transmission among thousands of migrant workers at factories and dormitories owned and run by Top Glove, a large Malaysian company that manufactures rubber gloves, face masks, and other rubber products: at the time of writing, over 4,000 confirmed cases have been linked to Top Glove. In response, authorities announced tough new legislation imposing a hefty RM50,000 fine on employers for each foreign worker found to be living in overcrowded lodging that is inconducive to safe distancing measures (*The Straits Times*, 2020b). The government also announced that they would be rolling out mass testing to 1.7 million migrant workers nationwide. While this is a welcome move, it is unclear if testing will be extended to Malaysia's approximately 2 million undocumented migrant workers, who typically do not have access to resources like healthcare and government aid, and risk detention or deportation if they step forward.

For Myanmar, porous borders have created large gaps in the surveillance of irregular migrants and during the pandemic have been important transmission routes both into and out of the country. Since April 2020, Myanmar saw over 150,000 migrants returning from Thailand that overwhelmed (or circumvented) health checkpoints. The country's second outbreak is believed by health officials to have been imported into northern Rakhine from neighbouring Bangladesh, which houses nearly a million Rohingya refugees (Radio Free Asia, 2020). In early December, Thailand reported its latest COVID cluster after Thai migrant workers sneaked back across the border from Myanmar (Associated Foreign Press, 2020). A variety of informal settlements, many of which lack proper health facilities, pose the risk of not only large clusters, but also of more severe outcomes. The country's different, protracted conflicts have created internally displaced persons (IDP) camps where hundreds of thousands reside in close proximity and many depending on external support for food and other essential supplies in several states. There were initial concerns that COVID-19 would course through the IDP camps in northern Rakhine that housed nearly half a million people, some of whom were displaced since 2012 due to communal violence, and more recently due to intensifying conflict. The jade mining region of Hpakant, home to over 300,000 camp-resident migrant workers with weak coverage of state services, has also seen a string of cases (Htwe, 2020a).

Although Singapore, an island city-state with no hinterland and tightly controlled borders, does not face the same access or border issues that affect Malaysia and Myanmar, it has had its share of vulnerable population challenges internally. Singapore is home to about 725,000 non-domestic migrant workers, many of whom are men from the South Asian subcontinent. An estimated 320,000 of these reside in worker dormitories, with the remaining workers living in temporary housing on construction sites and shipyards and in other residential premises. These dormitories tend to be densely packed, with many residents sharing a single room and shared facilities, including bathrooms and cooking areas. These close living conditions make physical distancing virtually impossible, thereby increasing the COVID-19 transmission risk. On 1 April, migrant workers accounted for only ten of 1,000 cases. By the end of the month, they comprised 89% of 15,600 cases in total; this was a prevalence rate over 50 times higher than that of the general population (Loong, 2020). Singaporean authorities moved quickly to contain the outbreak, pouring financial and manpower resources into efforts like mass swabbing and large-scale isolation of workers. However, it drew criticism for its outbreak management approach, with understaffing, disregard for living conditions in isolation, and lack of concern for workers' mental health identified as gaps (Ang, 2020). As of early December 2020, dormitories are no longer COVID-19 epicentres, but 54,000 of Singapore's 58,482 total confirmed cases remain linked to migrant worker dormitories (Yong, 2020).

Conclusion

Malaysia, Myanmar and Singapore's tackling of the COVID-19 pandemic show the wide gamut of tools and responses employed by countries on different rungs of the development ladder. While Singapore, as a highly-developed island city-state, has been among the few countries able to effectively control COVID-19 due to both preparedness and decisive response, it was still subject to critical blind spots and success may be challenging to replicate in differently resourced and governed settings. However, it serves as a benchmark on different criteria crucial for responding to ongoing and future public health emergencies. Malaysia and Myanmar's experiences with COVID-19 may be more in line with how the pandemic unfolds in other middle-income and developing countries. Their experiences also highlight the challenges and issues affecting COVID-19 response, from internal conflict in Myanmar to a full-blown political crisis in Malaysia. While effective vaccines have appeared on the horizon, how the COVID-19 pandemic continues to evolve in the three countries remains to be seen. Nonetheless, these countries' experiences serve to further enrich the evolving arsenal for pandemic preparedness and response.

Notes

1. Although a former British colony – first a province of India and then a Crown colony, Myanmar (formerly Burma) is not a member of the Commonwealth. However, it is included in this article as it broadens and enriches the study by enabling coverage of three Southeast Asian countries at different levels of economic development: Singapore, with one of the highest per capita GDP and GNI in the world; Malaysia, an upper middle-income country; and Myanmar, which just recently became classified as a lower middle-income country.
2. Malaysia increased its daily testing capacity from 1,000 tests per day in January 2020 to 38,000 tests per day in September 2020.

Disclosure statement

No potential conflict of interest was reported by the authors.

ORCID

Kyaw San Wai http://orcid.org/0000-0001-5212-0870
Wai Yee Krystal Khine http://orcid.org/0000-0001-7943-2866
Jane Mingjie Lim http://orcid.org/0000-0001-9017-4714
Pearlyn Hui Min Neo http://orcid.org/0000-0002-7797-8942
Rayner Kay Jin Tan http://orcid.org/0000-0002-9188-3368

Suan Ee Ong http://orcid.org/0000-0001-7365-9015

References

Ananthalakshmi, A., & Sipalan, J. (2020, March 17). *How mass pilgrimage at Malaysia mosque became coronavirus hotspot. Reuters.* https://www.reuters.com/article/us-health-coronavirus-malaysia-mosque-idUSKBN2142S4

Ang, H. M. (2020, September 12). *The long, challenging journey to bring COVID-19 under control in migrant worker dormitories. Channel News Asia.* https://www.channelnewsasia.com/news/singapore/in-focus-covid19-singapore-migrant-worker-dormitories-lockdown-13081210

Angel, H. (2020, November 11). *Private hospitals in Yangon and Mandalay to start treating COVID-19 patients. Myanmar Times.* https://www.mmtimes.com/news/private-hospitals-yangon-and-mandalay-start-treating-covid-19-patients.html

Associated Foreign Press. (2020, December 3). *Growing fears over Thai coronavirus cluster from Myanmar. Frontier Myanmar.* https://www.frontiermyanmar.net/en/growing-fears-over-thai-coronavirus-cluster-from-myanmar/

Awang, N. (2020). *Covid-19: Government may present plans for Phase 3 reopening in coming weeks, says Lawrence Wong. Today.* https://www.todayonline.com/singapore/covid-19-government-may-present-plans-phase-3-reopening-coming-weeks-says-lawrence-wong

Beech, H. (2020a, March 20). 'None of us have a fear of Corona': The faithful at an outbreak's center. *New York Times.* https://www.nytimes.com/2020/03/20/world/asia/coronavirus-malaysia-muslims-outbreak.html

Beech, H. (2020b, June 23). Singapore Calls for Elections Despite Pandemic. *The New York Times.* https://www.nytimes.com/2020/06/23/world/asia/singapore-elections-coronavirus.html

Bordier, M., & Roger, F. (2013). Zoonoses in South-East Asia: A regional burden, a global threat. *Animal Health Research Reviews, 14*(1), 40–67. https://doi.org/10.1017/S1466252313000017

Bunyan, J. (2020, September 22). *Putrajaya says no quarantine for voters returning from Sabah; Covid-19-positive cases not allowed to vote. Malay Mail.* https://www.malaymail.com/news/malaysia/2020/09/22/putrajaya-says-no-quarantine-for-voters-returning-from-sabah-covid-19-posit/1905556

CGTN. (2020, September 2). *China vows to prioritize Myanmar in sharing COVID-19 vaccine.* https://news.cgtn.com/news/2020-09-02/China-vows-to-prioritize-Myanmar-in-sharing-COVID-19-vaccine-TsEetIqmAw/index.html

Channel News Asia. (2020, November 28). *30% of Malaysians expected to be vaccinated against COVID-19 next year: PM Muhyiddin.* https://www.channelnewsasia.com/news/asia/covid-19-malaysia-vaccine-30-per-cent-population-muhyiddin-13657684

Chaudhury, D. R. (2020, October 23). *India gives priority on availability of anti Covid vaccines for Myanmar.* India Times. https://economictimes.indiatimes.com/news/politics-and-nation/india-gives-priority-on-availability-of-anti-covid-vaccines-for-myanmar/articleshow/78834600.cms?from=mdr

Chong, C., & Begum, S. (2020, December 7). *Phase 3 unlikely by end of year unless more use TRaceTogether, experts say. Straits Times.* https://www.straitstimes.com/singapore/phase-3-unlikely-by-end-of-year-unless-more-use-tracetogether-experts

Durgahyeni, M. (2019). *Budget 2020's health allocation not enough, analysts say.* https://codeblue.galencentre.org/2019/10/16/budget-2020s-health-allocation-not-enough-analysts-say/

Htwe, Z. Z. (2020a, September 29) *Yangon health official vows 'all-out battle' against COVID-19. Irrawaddy.* https://www.irrawaddy.com/specials/myanmar-covid-19/yangon-health-official-vows-battle-covid-19.html

Htwe, Z. Z. (2020b, October 20). *Myanmar's bustling jade hub under Covid-19 lockdown. Irrawaddy.* https://www.irrawaddy.com/news/burma/myanmars-bustling-jade-hub-covid-19-lockdown.html

International Labour Organization, ILO. (2020). *Assessment study on the skills of returned Myanmar migrants.* https://www.lift-fund.org/download/file/fid/6151

Jaipragas, B. (2020). *In Malaysia, questions over minister's small fine for coronavirus quarantine breach. South China Morning Post.* https://www.scmp.com/week-asia/politics/article/3098451/malaysia-questions-over-ministers-small-fine-coronavirus

Khor, S. (2019, October 23). *Budget 2020: More for healthcare with some missed opportunitie. The Star.* https://www.thestar.com.my/opinion/columnists/vital-signs/2019/10/23/budget-2020-more-for-healthcare-with-some-missed-opportunities

KPMG. (2020). *Malaysia: Government and institution measures in response to COVID-19.* https://home.kpmg/xx/en/home/insights/2020/04/malaysia-government-and-institution-measures-in-response-to-covid.html

Lim, V. W., Lim, R. L., Soh, A. S. E., Tan, M. X., Othman, N. B., Dickens, S. B., Thein, T. L., Lwin, M. O., Ong, R. T. H., Leo, Y. S., Lee, V. J., and Chen, M. I. C. (2020). Government trust, perceptions of COVID-19 and behaviour change: Cohort surveys, Singapore. *Bulletin of the World Health Organization.* Online first. Article ID BLT.20.269142. https://www.who.int/bulletin/online_first/BLT.20.269142.pdf?ua=1

Lin, R., Lee, T., & Lye, D. (2020). From SARS to COVID-19: The Singapore journey. *Medical Journal of Australia, 212*(11), 497–502.e491. https://doi.org/10.5694/mja2.50623

Loong, S. (2020, May 5). *Who is responsible for Singapore's migrant workers and why does it matter? Academia SG.* https://www.academia.sg/academic-views/who-is-responsible-for-singapores-migrant-workers-and-why-does-it-matter/

Malay Mail. (2020a, 26 September). *Sabah election kicks off with voters in full compliance with Covid-19 SOP.* https://www.malaymail.com/news/malaysia/2020/09/26/sabah-election-kicks-off-with-voters-in-full-compliance-with-covid-19-sop/1906850

Malay Mail. (2020b, November 22). *Communications Ministry to ramp up COVID-19 communication initiatives to prevent misinformation, 'trust deficit' in govt agencies.* https://www.malaymail.com/news/malaysia/2020/11/22/communications-ministry-to-ramp-up-covid-19-communication-initiatives-to-pr/1924994

Ministry of Finance Malaysia. (2019). *Speech text - Opening remark by minister of finance 2020 budget focus group meeting 3R approach to government healthcare.* https://www.treasury.gov.my/index.php/en/gallery-activities/speech/item/5483-speech-text-opening-remark-by-minister-of-finance-2020-budget-focus-group-meeting-3r-approach-to-government-healthcare.html#:~:text=Between%202010%20and%202018%2C%20the,a%20total%20allocation%20of%20RM28.

Ministry of Health and Sports, Myanmar. (2020). *Information to be aired in Rakhine and Bengali languages on Ma Yu FM and regional media (in Burmese).* https://mohs.gov.mm/page/10978

Ministry of Health, Malaysia. (2020). *COVID-19 Malaysia dashboard.* http://covid-19.moh.gov.my/

Moe, M. (2020, March 25). *Myanmar Speaker rejects call to summon military-majority security council to address COVID-19.* Irrawaddy. https://www.irrawaddy.com/news/burma/myanmar-speaker-rejects-call-summon-military-majority-security-council-address-covid-19.html

Myanmar News Agency. (2020, November 5). *MoLIP discusses distribution of COVID-19 medical devices for 2020 General election. Global New Light of Myanmar.* https://www.gnlm.com.mm/molip-discusses-distribution-of-covid-19-medical-devices-for-2020-general-election/

Naing, S. (2020, September 24). *Myanmar's 'maximum containment' COVID plan pushed to brink as virus surges. Reuters.* https://www.reuters.com/article/us-health-coronavirus-myanmar-idUSKCN26F0ZY

Povera, A., & Chan, D. (2020, June 7). *RMCO: Interstate travel allowed overseas travel not yet. New Straits Times.* https://www.nst.com.my/news/nation/2020/06/598714/rmco-interstate-travel-allowed-overseas-travel-not-yet

Radio Free Asia. (2020, October 6). *Myanmar's effort to trace COVID-19 spread treads on sensitive territory. Radio Free ASia.* https://www.rfa.org/english/news/myanmar/covid-19-spread-10062020174513.html

Ravindran, A. (2020, November 6). *Government slashes 2021 medical, public health budgets Amid Covid crisis. Code Blue.* https://codeblue.galencentre.org/2020/11/06/government-slashes-2021-medical-public-health-budgets-amid-covid-crisis/

The Straits Times. (2020a, October 4). *Covid-19: Sabah imposes strict conditions before allowing entry into state. The Straits Times.* https://www.straitstimes.com/asia/se-asia/covid-19-sabah-imposes-strict-conditions-before-allowing-entry-into-state

The Straits Times. (2020b, November 28). *Malaysia industries in shock as govt threatens to impose stiff fines on poor migrant lodgings. The Straits Times.* https://www.straitstimes.com/asia/se-asia/malaysia-industries-in-shock-as-govt-threatens-to-impose-stiff-fines-on-poor-migrant

Tan, A. (2020, December 1). *Moderna seeking HSA approval for use of its Covid-19 vaccine in Singapore. Straits Times.* https://www.straitstimes.com/singapore/health/moderna-seeking-approval-for-use-of-its-covid-19-vaccine-in-singapore

Tan, V. (2020, November 18). *Sabah's Batu Sapi by-election postponed as Malaysian king declares emergency for the parliamentary constituency. Channel News Asia.* https://www.channelnewsasia.com/news/asia/sabah-batu-sapi-by-election-postponed-malaysia-king-emergency-13585910

Tang, K. H. D. (2020). Movement control as an effective measure against Covid-19 spread in Malaysia: An overview. *Journal of Public Health*, 1–4. Advance online publication. https://doi.org/10.1007%2Fs10389-020-01316-w

Teo, J. (2020, November 28). *S'pore has no need to rely on one Covid-19 vaccine with several promising candidatesin the race. Straits Times.* https://www.straitstimes.com/singapore/health/no-need-to-rely-on-one-covid-19-vaccine-0

Tun, T. (2020, September 27). *COVID-19 Crisis: We will recover and build back better! Myanmar Digital News.* https://www.mdn.gov.mm/en/covid-19-crisis-we-will-recover-and-build-back-better

Wong, C. M. L. (2020). The paradox of trust: Perceived risk and public compliance during the COVID-19 pandemic in Singapore. *Journal of Risk Research*, *23*(7–8), 1021–1030. https://doi.org/10.1080/13669877.2020.1756386

World Health Organization. (2020, September 4). *Universal health coverage and COVID-19 preparedness & response in Malaysia.* https://www.who.int/malaysia/news/detail/04-09-2020-universal-health-coverage-and-covid-19-preparedness-response-in-malaysia

Yi, H., Ng, S., Farwin, A., Low, A., Chang, C., & Lim, J. (2020). Health equity considerations in COVID-19: Geospatial network analysis of the COVID-19 outbreak in the migrant population in Singapore. *Journal of Travel Medicine, taaa159.* https://doi.org/10.1093/jtm/taaa159

Yong, M. (2020, October 13). *Timeline: No new COVID-19 case in Singapore's dormitories for the first time in 6 months. Channel News Asia.* https://www.channelnewsasia.com/news/singapore/covid-19-cases-singapore-dormitory-zero-six-months-13271976

Impacts of COVID-19 in the Commonwealth Caribbean: key lessons

Jessica Byron, Jacqueline Laguardia Martinez, Annita Montoute and Keron Niles

ABSTRACT
COVID-19 has further weakened the fragile socio-economic fabric of the Commonwealth Caribbean (CC). Economies have been stifled by 'lockdowns', and by a global decline in travel and tourism. The result has been higher levels of indebtedness, unemployment and psychological stress, disproportionately affecting vulnerable populations throughout the region. Despite their limited size and resources, CC states have sought to support business and individuals alike, stimulate economic activity and preserve livelihoods. In this article, the authors acknowledge multilateral and regional policy responses, and argue that the present scenario offers opportunities to deepen functional cooperation and build resilience.

Introduction

Since the confirmation of the first case of COVID-19 in the Americas, there has been an epidemiological trend of increasing cases in the region. The evolution of the pandemic has been accompanied by misinformation, excessive information, and by deepening gender, ethnic and economic inequalities (Basile, 2020). The fragilities of public health systems in the region have been exposed and for most of the second half of 2020, the Americas have been considered the epicentre of the pandemic.

This article on the impact of COVID-19 in the Commonwealth Caribbean (CC),[1] a small part of the Americas, records the territories' extreme fragilities as well as their efforts to construct resilient responses to the crisis by strategic use of domestic, regional and global governance, cooperation and diplomacy.[2] Our analysis emphasises the significance of their geographies and (relative) remoteness, governance implications associated with small size, and the stark vulnerability and restructuring imperatives that confront export-oriented economies heavily dependent on tourism, air and maritime transport, financial services, remittances and commodities (including fossil fuels) in the contemporary era (Table 1). Currently, there are grim projections about the economic consequences of the pandemic for most Caribbean economies (ECLAC, 2020b; OECS, 2020a).

The case study portrays a relatively successful first phase of containing disease spread and fatalities despite limited health infrastructure and resources (Figures 1 and 2). It also

Table 1. Economic impact of tourism in CC countries. 2019.

	Total Contribution to GDP		Total Contribution to Employment	
CC countries	Percent (%)	US$ millions	Share (%)	Jobs
Antigua and Barbuda	44.7	1.477	44.7	16.654
Bahamas	40.3	5.273	48.1	102.505
Barbados	36.2	1.693	36.4	47.829
Belize	44.7	879	38.9	63.410
Dominica	38	200	34.7	12.202
Grenada	55.8	708	51.6	27.179
Jamaica	34.7	5.467	31.5	388.767
St. Kitts and Nevis	62.6	670	60.2	15.324
St. Lucia	43	1.153	43	34.297
St. Vincent and the Grenadines	46.2	385	42.7	18.901
Trinidad and Tobago	7.8	2.361	9.9	62.067

Source: (Dukharan, 2020), p. 6

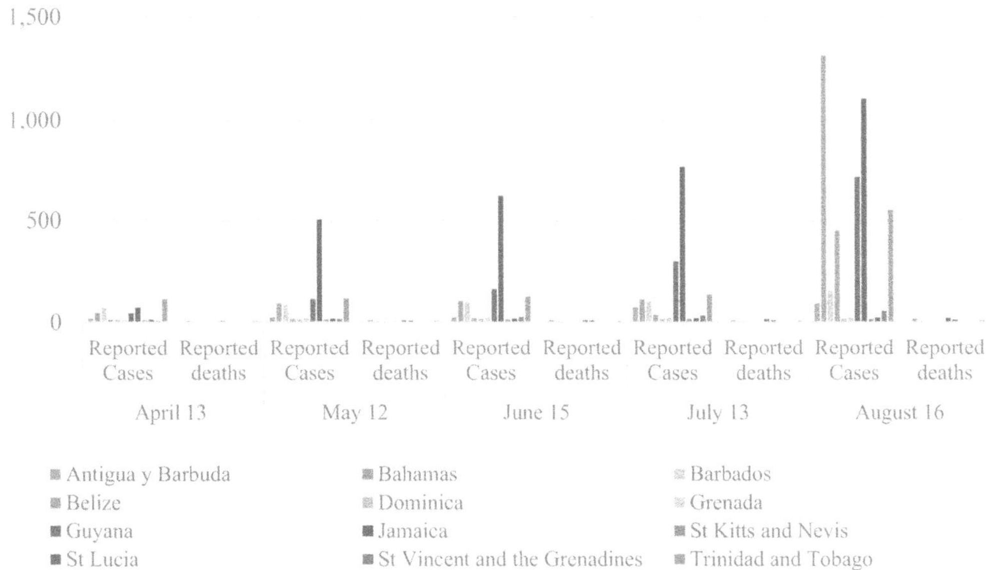

Figure 1. Confirmed COVID-19 cases in CC countries (April-August 2020). Source: Coronavirus Resource Centre at John Hopkins University.

captures the challenges of the second phase of increased COVID-19 infections while reopening national borders and relaunching economic and social activity. It demonstrates advantages and drawbacks of the geographical characteristics of these Small Island Developing States (SIDS), and how they have sought to leverage such factors.[3]

The CC is part of a larger Caribbean space, strongly attached to the geopolitical and geo-economic poles of the Americas. Its experience of the pandemic has been influenced by its location and developments in the surrounding geopolitical space. COVID-19 has highlighted the risks inherent in the region's manner of integration into the global economy, it has precipitated technological changes and major societal adjustments and it will compound the region's economic challenges. The pandemic has reconfigured

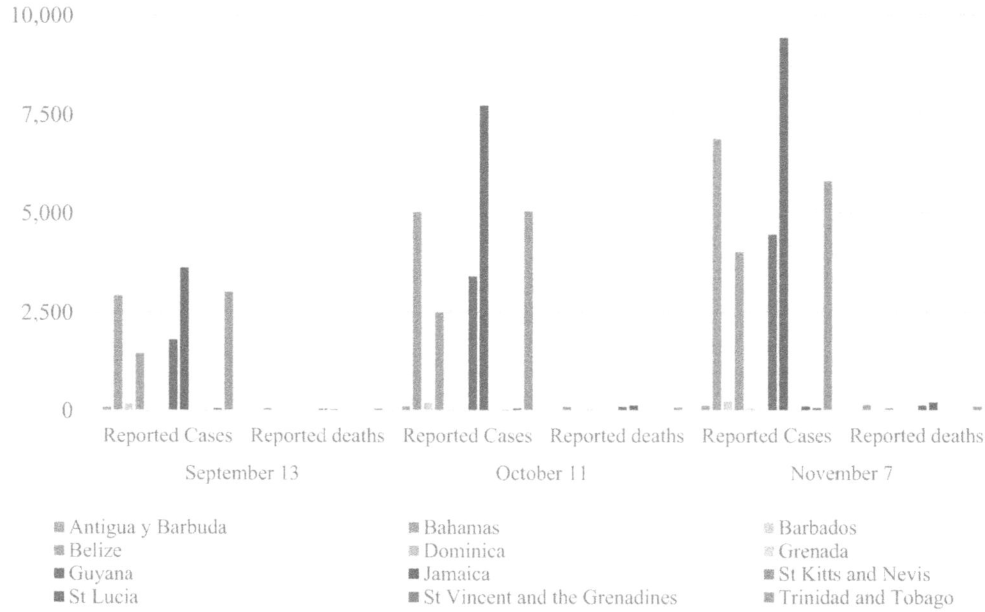

Figure 2. Confirmed COVID-19 cases in CC countries (September-November 2020). Source: Coronavirus Resource Centre at John Hopkins University.

regional and national governance in numerous ways, and has influenced the processes and outcomes of national elections in at least three CC polities in 2020.

The article gives an overview of the economic, social and political impacts of COVID-19 in CC states and the national and regional responses. The discussion identifies local and external drivers of public policy, and explores the dynamics of governance processes in pandemic conditions. The final section highlights significant outcomes and emphasises the lessons of COVID-19 for the Caribbean in terms of social, economic and political restructuring.

Economic impact and policy responses

The negative economic impacts associated with COVID-19 for CC territories are linked to the region's high dependence on tourism and remittances, economic openness and limited resources. Cumulative weak economic growth, high debt and unemployment rates exacerbate the gloomy scenario, particularly for those CC countries that are among the most heavily tourism-dependent economies in the world (Mooney & Zegorra, 2020). UNICEF (2020) estimates an average loss of 27% of formal sector employment in the Eastern Caribbean which would be somewhat lower in countries with higher proportions of agricultural employment.

Most CC countries are trapped in high public debt largely because of their constant need for funds to repair structural damage from extreme meteorological events. ECLAC (2020a:5) points out that despite achieving primary surpluses averaging 0.8% of GDP in the past decade, government budgets show overall annual deficits averaging 2.5% of GDP. The pandemic has increased financing challenges, which include health service expenditure and social support. These additional costs combined with less revenue generation will further constrict fiscal space and increase debt. Given the widespread adverse economic impacts of COVID-19, traditional donors may be less willing and able to enter into development cooperation agreements and offer assistance to developing countries.

Leveraging support from multilateral development agencies is therefore likely to be crucial to the process of restructuring and rebuilding. CC states have mobilised resources from International Financial Institutions (IFIs) such as the International Monetary Fund (IMF). Within this context, minimising the cost of such debt while limiting the impact of lending conditionalities on national sovereignty is likely to be a priority concern of policy makers in the short term. In the second quarter of 2020, the IMF, through its Rapid Financing Instrument, the Extended Fund Facility or Special Drawing Rights facility, made emergency funding available to seven CC states in amounts ranging from US$520 million for Jamaica to US$14 million for Dominica (International Monetary Fund (IMF), 2020). Likewise, the Interamerican Development Bank is facilitating a US$34 million loan to Guyana for COVID-19 pandemic purposes (GECOM, 2020).

COVID-19 negatively affects the investment risk profiles of small, open, environmentally vulnerable nations. This has implications for commercial insurance and overall investment costs in the CC which may rise if the costs of financial and other services required to support such investments increase due to external shocks. One example of adverse impacts is the suspension of CC airline services in July and September 2020 representing a major blow to regional connectivity and to employment (Baptiste, 2020; Nanton, 2020).

For economies based on oil and gas exports, COVID-19 has dramatically decreased the demand for energy, due to reduced international and domestic travel. With an excess supply of oil on the international market, prices which have been trending downward since 2015 are not expected to significantly rebound soon. COVID-19 has therefore exacerbated the impacts of decreased government revenues that were already being experienced by CC energy exporters. Trinidad and Tobago illustrate this trend. An increase in the country's deficit spending has accompanied the decreased contributions of the energy sector to GDP. The budget deficit has increased from approximately TTD 3 billion in 2015 to approximately TTD 17 billion in 2020 (Imbert, 2020). Dependence on the national Heritage and Stabilisation Fund (HSF) was heightened by the global pandemic as it served as a key source of financing for a government stimulus programme that included expanded social assistance, income support programmes and rental assistance for households affected by job loss or salary reduction. COVID-19 accounted for the withdrawal of US$900 million from the HSF between May and August 2020 (Dhanpaul, 2020).

Simultaneously, the scenario brought about by the pandemic (with respect to energy prices) is likely to dampen economic growth in both Guyana and Suriname, although an increase in the international price of gold in 2020 (Business Insider, 2020; Simoes & Hidalgo, 2011) should help to keep their extractive economies afloat. In the case of Guyana, priority must also be given to restoring social and economic stability after recent election-related unrest and violence.

The pandemic has affected production across most CC sectors since health policies designed to contain the spread of the virus restricted the movement of people through quarantines, social isolation and border closures (Economic Commission for Latin America and the Caribbean (ECLAC), 2020a). In the ensuing economic downturn, companies have suffered from declining revenue, credit difficulties and insolvency risks. Labour market conditions have deteriorated. CC economies (minus Guyana) are expected to contract by 7.9% overall in 2020 (Economic Commission for Latin America and the Caribbean (ECLAC), 2020b, pp. 7–8).[4]

Throughout the Caribbean, informal sectors often rely on formal sector activity. Persons in these economic spheres are generally uninsured individuals or irregular migrants without access to official business support channels. They are highly exposed to market shocks and have suffered disproportionately from the economic contraction. To cope with the negative economic impacts, CC countries reacted quickly to the initial stage of the crisis. Public resources like stimulus packages and the provision of baskets of goods were channelled to the health sector and used to protect households, support production capacity and employees, and prevent economic collapse (Economic Commission for Latin America and the Caribbean (ECLAC), 2020a). Such measures did not ameliorate conditions for the informal sector.

These measures were implemented to 'preserve bank liquidity, support commerce and address public and private debt' (Economic Commission for Latin America and the Caribbean (ECLAC), 2020a, p. 13). Governments relied on fiscal measures to redirect budgets and introduced tax relief and exemption measures. Economic provisions were accompanied by social protection initiatives to cover vulnerable persons (Economic Commission for Latin America and the Caribbean (ECLAC), 2020a). Justin Ram (2020) has argued that there is need to expand and innovate financial services within the Caribbean by creating new instruments to reach underserved, low-income groups, and encouraging entrepreneurship, perhaps through micro-finance facilities. Such instruments could strengthen financial literacy and create opportunities for those in the informal sector to be integrated within the formal economy.

Some CC countries have been better positioned than others to mitigate the economic impacts with counter-cyclical fiscal and monetary stimuli. However, most solutions have been at least partially debt-financed and this represents a major problem for an already highly indebted region (Dukharan, 2020). The effects in each country vary according to the preceding economic conditions and production structures. For countries like Jamaica, recently emerged from IMF restructuring programmes, COVID-19 has dealt a crushing blow to economic recovery efforts. In spite of CC measures, the pandemic is expected to lead to the most severe economic contraction since records began in 1900 (Economic Commission for Latin America and the Caribbean (ECLAC), 2020a). CC economies will be negatively affected by the following phenomena:

- Collapse of global trade, estimated at between 13% and 32% in 2020 (Economic Commission for Latin America and the Caribbean (ECLAC), 2020a, p. 7).
- The global negative impact on services, especially entertainment and tourism, with an estimated drop in 2020 tourist arrivals of between 58% and 78% (United Nations Conference on Trade and Development (UNCTAD), 2020, p. 21). The hard-hit Caribbean tourism sector accounts for 15.5% of GDP and employs approximately 2.4 million people (Economic Commission for Latin America and the Caribbean (ECLAC), 2020a, p. 11). Recovery depends on how and when borders open.

- Commodity exporters like Guyana and Trinidad and Tobago will suffer from an estimated 20% to 30% fall in energy prices (Comisión Económica para América Latina y el Caribe (CEPAL), 2020).
- Increased financial vulnerabilities are associated with massive capital outflows in emerging markets and the depreciation of domestic currencies against the U.S. dollar. Financial volatility – measured by the CBOE Volatility Index – rose to all-time highs in mid-March (Comisión Económica para América Latina y el Caribe (CEPAL), 2020).
- Remittance flows to Latin America and the Caribbean globally are estimated to contract by 15% in 2020 (Economic Commission for Latin America and the Caribbean (ECLAC), 2020a).

Social impact and policy responses

Many social impacts of the pandemic stem from economic closure and its consequences. Other repercussions emanate from restrictions on social activities and networks which traditionally provided supporting buffers. Preliminary evidence shows that poorer sections of the society disproportionally bear the health and economic impacts of the pandemic. The homeless, those without access to running water, migrants, displaced persons, the elderly, persons with disabilities, indigenous peoples and youth face greater risks. Women and children also suffer disproportionately (OECS, 2020a).

The pandemic has exposed the inadequacies of health care systems in the region. Governments have responded by increasing expenditure on health care in many CC countries. Antigua and Barbuda and St. Kitts and Nevis increased their health care budget by 0.5% of their GDP. In Guyana, the allocation made for each of the health and education sectors was 15% of GDP. Some countries provided concessions on the import of PPE and relevant medical supplies to make them more affordable to the public as in the case of Jamaica, St. Kitts and Nevis, St, Vincent and the Grenadines, Trinidad and Tobago (IMF, 2020). Countries have largely prioritised containment measures to avoid overwhelming the limited resources of the health sector (OECS, 2020a). The case of Trinidad and Tobago is worth highlighting as it was ranked number one in its response to the early stages of the pandemic on March 12th, 2020, in a report by the University of Oxford. The success of the health system was said to have resulted from an approach which was well-coordinated, collaborative and evidence based (Hunte et al., 2020). Other countries had few cases and a low or zero mortality rate including St Lucia, St. Vincent and the Grenadines, Dominica and St. Kitts and Nevis.[5] Nevertheless, the pandemic will stimulate much-needed reform and improved capacity in this sphere (OECS, 2020a). Several signs point in this direction. Many countries have increased their health budget and local manufacturing of medical equipment and supplies has been bolstered in countries like Trinidad and Tobago. The recognition that coordinated efforts, timely statistical data and other relevant information are critical to successfully navigating health crises means that it will not be business as usual in the health sector in a post-COVID environment. Finally, the pandemic has highlighted to health authorities and the general population the need to prioritise preventative health care and perhaps enforce related measures.

The education sector faces challenges because of school closures coupled with the move to online teaching delivery (OECS, 2020b). In Jamaica, approximately 31,656 teachers and 627,000 students have been impacted by the closure of school (UNESCO, 2020). This has precipitated a dramatic increase in the use of information and communications technology in the education sector, and major disruptions in teaching and learning (OECS, 2020b). Although computer and internet access is high in the Caribbean, 40% of users access it outside the home with only about 50% of households having a computer for home use. Issues around internet coverage and reliability exacerbate the challenges of online teaching and learning (USAID and UNICEF, 2020). CC countries have reported challenges including limited capacity (technical and financial resources) to transit to online learning, the absence of a harmonised approach to enact solutions, negative impact on students' emotional wellbeing, heightened insecurity and vulnerability and disproportionate access for economically disadvantaged students. Children who depend on school feeding programmes may have experienced reduced nutrition with school closures,[6] and there has also been a reduction in the time dedicated to learning (OECS Commission, 2020a, 2020b; Flowers, 2020; UNICEF, 2020; USAID and UNESCO, 2020), in many cases, limited parental support with learning due to low education levels (Flowers, 2020) and disruption of regional certification examinations.

At the same time, the disruption has fuelled responses which could have long-term positive impacts. In its strategic response plan, the OECS proposes to harmonise policy responses among member states, make the transition to a digital education system, strengthen safety nets for students and promote engagement to coordinate interventions. Several countries have embarked on online and blended learning training for teachers during COVID-19 and beyond. Teaching and learning digital technology have been launched or expanded in various countries. Some countries have increased internet connectivity for schools and provided or expanded access to electronic devices for students. These developments will expand the digitalisation of teaching and learning and increase ICT literacy in the CC, which should have spillover beneficial effects for other sectors of the economy (OECS Commisssion, 2020b).

Policy responses to cushion the impact on the most vulnerable have included measures to boost employment in labour-intensive sectors like construction. The preceding section has outlined fiscal interventions aimed at social protection, unemployment benefits and salary support packages. It should be noted that with the onset of the pandemic and new poverty projections, it was estimated that existing social assistance programmes would only cover approximately 11% of the most vulnerable in Antigua and Barbuda and St. Lucia, approximately 30% in Trinidad and Tobago, 43% and 45% in St Kitts and Nevis and Grenada respectively and 76% in St. Vincent and the Grenadines (USAID and UNICEF, 2020). Thus the pandemic revealed the inadequacies of existing social assistance programmes in a crisis. For example, in Jamaica, the US$73 million allocated to the COVID Allocation of Resources for Employees (CARE) programme proved to be insufficient early in the pandemic.

While devising new emergency measures, many CC governments expanded existing programmes to meet demands arising from the adverse pandemic effects. Some examples include Antigua's COVID-19 Government Assistance Food Voucher

Programme which is an expansion of the GAP (Social Safety Net) programme (UNICEF and UN Women Eastern Caribbean, 2020a; IMF, 2020). St Vincent and the Grenadines expanded social safety net programmes and St. Kitts and Nevis provided additional support for its poverty alleviation programme (IMF 2020). Grenada expanded the government employment programmes while Barbados expanded unemployment benefits to self-employed workers, vertically expanded National Assistance payments and broadened horizontal coverage under the National Assistance programme (UNICEF, 2020).

However, the IDB's prognosis is that despite their mitigating effect, 'safety nets coverage are also a source of inefficiencies in the public spending system … leakage is significant' (Beuermann et al., 2020, para. 6). Some administration and implementation difficulties that were experienced suggest that states should guard against inventing too many new programmes in times of crisis and focus on channelling support through existing programmes (Mera, 2020, p. 14).

The pandemic has highlighted the dangers of neglecting social development and underscored the need to address development holistically. There is particular need to focus on vulnerable groups by boosting and maintaining social protection measures, supporting and advancing the rights to health, safety, and dignity for persons with disabilities (OECS, 2020a) and the elderly. Civil society organisations' participation has also proven to be vital as they are well-placed to link health to broader development challenges and to facilitate bottom–up solutions. In general, civil society actors have a long track record of supporting or complementing the state in delivering health services to the citizenry. They do so independently or in partnership with the state. Scholars argue that civil society actors play a vital role in the sphere of health (Doyle & Patel, 2008; Smith et al., 2016; Storeng & Puyvalle, 2018). Smith et al. (2016) argue that civil society can make strong moral arguments to push governments into action, foster collaboration with other sectors to support health, innovate new policy alternatives and promote legitimacy of health initiatives and institutions. They may also strengthen health systems, foster accountability, guard against the pursuit of commercial interests in health and elevate rights-based approaches. Their role has been recognised in international documents which acknowledge health as a basic human right and emphasise participation of the individual and community in health policy design as a civic right and duty (PAHO and WHO, 2017). UNAIDS Caribbean has urged Caribbean governments to include relevant CSOs in the decision-making and planning processes for meeting the needs of their most vulnerable populations and to provide support to these groups (UNAIDS, 2020).

The CC COVID response has been largely dominated by the state with CSOs calling for inclusion in some countries. For instance, Civil Society Bahamas called for CSO inclusion in designing the national plan for country's future (McKenzie, 2020), while the St. Lucia Bar Association lamented the lack of public consultation on the COVID-19 (Prevention & Control) Bill, 2020 (CNG News, 2020). However, there are cases of state-civil society collaboration. In Guyana, several CSOs are engaged in work of National Emergency Operations Centre, part of the national framework to combat the virus (GECOM, 2020). Other examples include the Women's Institute for Alternative Development in Trinidad and Tobago launching a mask production project funded by the private sector (Attzs, 2020) and GROOTS

Trinidad and Tobago provision of meals to affected persons and advice to citizens trying to navigate government assistance schemes (UNAIDS, 2020). Some CSOs have sought to insert their agenda in governments' responses. The Healthy Caribbean Coalition (HCC) urged governments to take urgent action to protect persons living with NCDs from COVID-19 (HCC, 2020), while the Cropper Foundation in Trinidad advocates linking health challenges to the environment and broader development agenda (LoopNews, 2020). The UWI Institute for Gender and Development Studies has campaigned for governments to provide better resources for CSOs providing safety and shelter for domestic violence victims, also critiquing the lack of gender expertise on the Trinidad and Tobago Post-COVID National Recovery Committee (The UWI St Augustine, 2020).

Caribbean electoral developments and the role of the state

COVID-19 struck in an extremely active electoral year for the Caribbean (McDonald, 2020). The International Institute for Democracy and Electoral Assistance (IDEA) notes an initial worldwide tendency in 2020 to postpone elections based on health and electoral integrity concerns. This changed as appropriate organisational responses were developed. IDEA's survey also shows declines in voter turnout in 2020, compared to the statistics for 2008–2019 (International IDEA, 2020). Except for the outlier state of Guyana, both observations are relevant to the Caribbean. COVID-19 served to bring forward some national polls, while others were delayed due to the states of emergency imposed in selected countries.[7] The virus dramatically eroded the social and economic context in which elections were being held, shifting the primary concerns of the electorate, the discourse of the candidates, conduct of campaigns and polling.

During 2020, eleven Caribbean states or territories have held elections, among them six CC states.[8] While four incumbent administrations (Jamaica, St. Kitts and Nevis, St. Vincent and the Grenadines and Trinidad and Tobago) were returned to office, new administrations elected in Belize and the South American Caribbean may influence evolution in national and regional policy-making.

The circumstances of the Guyanese election were distinct from all others. Historical socio-political forces coupled with the high economic stakes at play set the stage for this poll to degenerate into a bitter, long drawn-out stalemate, creating an additional crisis on the regional agenda. During the pandemic, CARICOM member states, regional organisations and civil society devoted considerable time and resources to facilitate a peaceful, democratic transition of power in Guyana (Larocque, 2020). This finally happened on 2 August 2020.[9]

Other elections were affected by the pandemic in various ways. Some electoral debates were cancelled. Campaigning was modified for social distancing, virtual engagement with voters outweighed the usual large assemblies and house to house campaigns. Nonetheless, there were reports of post-election infection spikes in Trinidad and Jamaica (Figure 3) (Allen, 2020; *The Economist*, 2020; Robinson, 2020; Stabroek News, 2020a). Closed borders in St. Kitts and Trinidad prevented voters overseas from returning home to vote. Electoral observation was also reduced. While observation took place in St. Kitts, St Vincent and Belize, neither Commonwealth nor

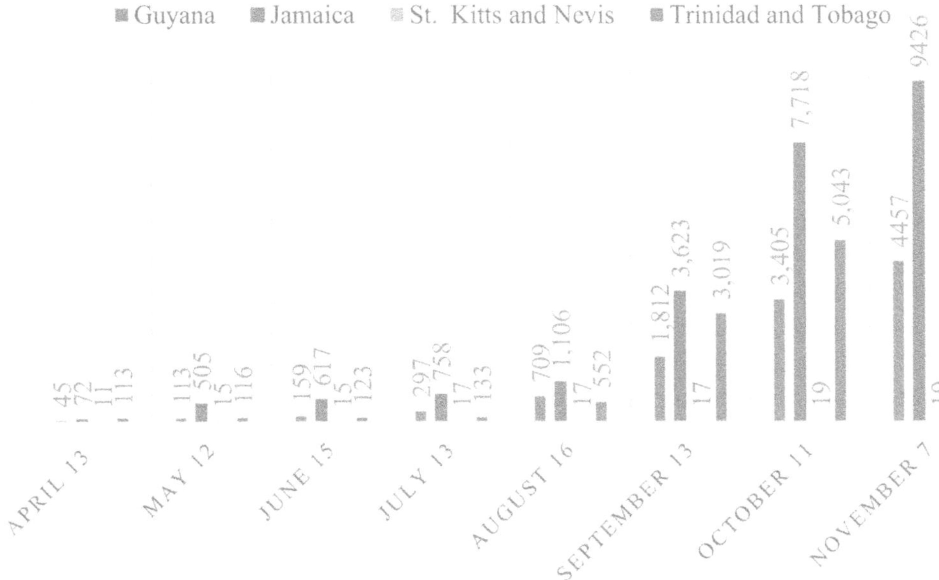

Figure 3. Confirmed COVID-19 cases in CC countries that held elections (November 7). Source: Coronavirus Resource Centre at John Hopkins University.

CARICOM observers were present in Trinidad and Tobago due to the financial and quarantine constraints of organising missions (Taitt, 2020). Finally, in Jamaica, there was a historically low voter turnout of 37% with public health fears cited as one possible factor (Thompson, 2020). Voter turnout was highest in the three CARICOM countries where governments were replaced (ranging from 70% to 82%) and ranged from 67% to 58% in all other jurisdictions except for Jamaica.[10]

COVID-19 influenced electoral discourse in other ways. It broadened voters' yardstick for assessing leadership (*Sunday Express*, 2020; Wyss, 2020). In addition to the continued importance of longstanding societal concerns – the economy, citizen security, corruption – the ratings of some incumbent administrations may have also been affected by public perceptions of their management of the pandemic, social protection issues and the economy. Some governments, possibly anticipating the onset of sharply deteriorating economic conditions, brought elections forward, and may have benefited from favourable public health results during the first phase of COVID-19.

During COVID-19, prominent women, including Barbados's Prime Minister, have supported global humanitarian initiatives and have been portrayed as good practice examples of female leadership (Rodriguez, 2020; Wilkinson, 2020). However, CC electoral results during this period give mixed messages about women's political representation in the Caribbean. Although Jamaica elected its highest ever number of women parliamentarians, there are only five female ministers out of 28, while the St. Kitts and Nevis cabinet features only two women among 11 ministers. The Trinidad and Tobago administration almost reached parity with nine female ministers out of 21. Guyana has an electoral quota system and 25 of its 65 parliamentarians are female.[11]. Belize has two women ministers and three female parliamentarians while St. Vincent has no female ministers. Nonetheless, all these national elections saw an increased presence of new and more youthful political representatives. COVID-19 has highlighted longstanding Caribbean gender inequality issues, especially the prevalence of domestic violence and the pressures faced by women struggling with child care and income generation during lockdowns and school closure. It remains to be seen how these issues will be addressed in the next iteration of national and regional politics.

Globally, COVID-19 has precipitated a major rethink of the state's role and priorities for state/societal relations. Casas-Zamora (2020) argues that effective governance systems and real institutional capacity to cope with crisis and uncertainty have emerged as essential requirements for the state, regardless of its form. ECLAC, UNDP and other multilateral agencies continue to highlight that socio-economic inequalities are major risk factors in the pandemic and exhort countries to build social resilience by focusing on the needs of their most vulnerable populations. The Caribbean has also been exhorted to sharpen its focus on environmental protection and sustainability and continue building resilience to natural disasters as key components of the rebuilding efforts in an environmentally sensitive and extremely climate-sensitive region (Economic Commission for Latin America and the Caribbean (ECLAC), 2020a,b). Environmental sustainability, along with social inclusiveness must be central components of the economic rebuilding process.

The foregoing discussions have underscored the extent to which public health security depends on partnership and consensus-building between state and society. Scholars have long suggested that characteristics of small-scale societies include high levels of social cohesion, frequency and informality of consultation among elites and the public, as well as the pervasive presence of government (Sutton, 2007). We contend that these characteristics, as well as historical experiences of coping with natural disasters were leveraged by CC states in confronting the political dimensions of COVID-19.

The pandemic elevated the portfolios of health, education and social protection, challenging the CC state to focus more on human security, and on transparent communication that engenders citizens' trust. Many states adjusted their practices in the areas of communication, law enforcement and to the extent possible, social protection. There is evidence of more structured government communication strategies and processes. Most CC states sought to break down administrative silos by appointing national coordinating committees comprising executive actors, public health and national security officials and featuring other key departments when necessary. Some countries also established national and/or regional recovery task forces to address the social and economic fallout of the pandemic. Communication strategies included frequent press conferences, public announcements and regular gazettes with updates on the epidemic and new government regulations, and extensive public education about the disease and health and safety protocols. Such measures were aimed both at educating and at neutralising the impact of misinformation.

Other more coercive actions concerned measures to restrict population mobility through shelter in place measures, curfews and national or localised economic lockdowns. Ten states, especially between March and June 2020, imposed national or localised states of emergency to enforce public compliance with prohibitions against the frequenting of bars, beaches and other recreational places. All countries temporarily banned religious gatherings. CC states closed their borders for varying durations and have since maintained public health-related border protocols. Many measures, although coordinated by the state, were policy recommendations from regional and global public health agencies, based on available scientific information. COVID-era governance has driven increased consultation with private sector and civil society entities in quest of proposals and feedback, and to generate greater acceptance of 'the new normal' by the population.

Issues that have generated public anxiety and critical debates on human rights and health security include the situation of nationals stranded abroad during national lockdowns and states' slow progress in formulating appropriate consular and other repatriation arrangements.[12] Another issue, with particular relevance to Trinidad and Tobago, and on which there are contending human rights and national security perspectives, concerns the state's responsibility to migrants and asylum seekers during the pandemic.[13] Other themes that arguably may surface in CC political debates in future include the adequacy of existing constitutional or legislative instruments in many CC states to respond flexibly to such emergencies, and the extent to which bipartisanship was drawn on as a resource available to CC states during national crises.

Regionalism: indispensable dimension of CC public action

'If ever there was a time that we understand the importance of these regional institutions, it is now' (Mottley, 2020).

In CC small states, regional cooperation has historically underpinned and bolstered limited national capacity through resource-pooling and coordinated responses. It has also been used to manage asymmetrical power relations. CC regionalism often gets critical reviews for having fallen short of its potential (Bishop & Payne, 2010; Byron, 2014; Girvan, 2010), although CARICOM is viewed as one of the hemisphere's most stable regional groupings. Indeed, a positive indication of CARICOM's maturity as a regional governance institution and the quality of its recent leadership is that regional governance processes have not faltered during the pandemic despite several national elections, the inevitable distractions of the electoral cycles, and occasional policy differences among governments in the handling of the crisis.

Caribbean regionalism has rested on two main drivers, political summitry and functional cooperation activities (Byron, 2016; Collins, 2008). In the case of CARICOM, both went into high gear during COVID-19 under the energetic chairmanship of Barbados PM Mottley (Bardouille, 2020; Knight & Reddy Srikanth, 2020). CARICOM has played a major role in managing the pandemic in the region by harmonising the responses and policies relating to COVID-19, pooling resources and representing the region's agenda in global and regional fora and in various bilateral and multilateral partner meetings.

Between February and July 2020, CARICOM Heads of Government held five formal meetings, several informal consultations, meetings of their executive Bureau and of the Council for Human and Social Development (COHSOD) (Larocque, 2020). Such intense caucusing was facilitated by advances in the use of videoconferencing technology which have profoundly changed the *modus operandi* of CC regional cooperation. Regional and global multilateral agencies joined forces to provide coordinated responses, expert advice and material resources in the areas of public health, border management, food security, transport and supply logistics, research data and financial support. They included Caribbean Public Health Agency, Caribbean Disaster and Emergency Management Agency, Caribbean Agricultural Research and Development Institute, Caribbean Development Bank, Implementing Agency for Crime and Security, The University of the West Indies, OECS and its agencies including the Eastern Caribbean Central Bank, PAHO and the World Health Organisation.

CC states agreed in April 2020 on joint responses to the pandemic in public health, the regional economy and food security. They committed to strengthening the digital infrastructure for health, commerce and e-governance more generally. They agreed to adopt joint procurement procedures for medical supplies and personnel for COVID-19 (Caribbean Council, 2020a; CARICOM Secretariat, 2020). In May 2020, the Heads of Government agreed to consider a joint approach prepared by a regional inter-agency working group to open borders, negotiate with the cruise and airline industries and to reopen tourism and other economic sectors (Caribbean Council, 2020b, 2020c; CARICOM Secretariat, 2020). In September 2020, the Heads of Government agreed to initiate a regional travel bubble with CARPHA-recommended operational procedures and eligibility criteria. It was argued that Barbados and the OECS countries currently meet the criteria, other states may join later and this would stimulate air links and revive intraregional mobility and connectivity (Stabroek News, September 2020b). However, this proposal has not been implemented and regional mobility remains a major challenge at the end of 2020.

A substantial part of CARICOM's response has been implemented via CARPHA, the CC regional public health agency that has been in operation since 2013 and the region's collective means of effectively addressing the changing nature of public health challenges. CARPHA's key actions have included the coordination of a regional response; the issuing of situation reports and press releases to stakeholders; the preparation of travel, air and seaport guidelines; working with IMPACS on a Security Cluster for passenger tracking. Other crucial contributions have been the provision of COVID-19 testing services and regular laboratory updates, the tracking of COVID developments, and the training of CC health personnel (CARPHA, 2020; Interamerican Development Bank (IADB), 2020).

CC states harnessed their regional/interregional networks as platforms for greater diplomatic visibility and impact during the pandemic. CARICOM's coordinated use of multilateral diplomacy bore fruit first in the close working relationship with the WHO and PAHO and the committed scientific and technological support received from both agencies. Additionally, CARICOM, through the good offices of the WHO and the African members of the Africa Caribbean Pacific Group was added to the African Medical Supplies Platform, which guarantees supplies of COVID-19 medical equipment at competitive prices, another focus was their collective lobbying of the IFIs to consider the vulnerabilities of highly indebted middle-income developing countries, provide debt relief and relax the criteria for development assistance (CARICOM Secretariat, 2020). The Heads of Government also called for the lifting of sanctions on Venezuela and Cuba on humanitarian grounds, and lamented resource challenges being faced by the WHO (Caribbean Council 2020a). CARICOM's cooperation agreements with Cuba resulted in over 650 Cuban medical professionals being provided to the various CC states to reinforce local resources (MINREX, 2020). Bilateral diplomacy has garnered cooperation and support during the pandemic from many countries in the form of medical supplies, protection for stranded CARICOM nationals, and broader economic support. COVID-19 has undoubtedly galvanised CARICOM's capacity for a coordinated crisis response.

It has given a sharp reminder of the imperative for strong, effective Caribbean regional institutions. At the same time, events have also demonstrated the continuing limitations to the process, as attempts to coordinate border and economic reopening and to present a united front to significant sectors, like the travel industry, have faltered (Caribbean Council 2020b, 2020c). The acid test of the new regional impetus will come as economic crises deepen and national administrations risk becoming so engulfed in domestic challenges that regional integration and coordination are once again placed on the back burner.

Another avenue for regional cooperation has been provided by the Association of Caribbean States (ACS). ACS Foreign Relations and Health Ministers met in March 2020 to explore joint responses and strategies to address the pandemic. This was followed up by a meeting in April of ACS Founding Observers – Central American Integration System, CARICOM, Economic Commission for Latin America and the Caribbean, Latin American Economic System, Caribbean Tourism Organisation and Central American Integration System – to exchange experiences and ideas for a better regional coordination response. The ACS provides the perspective of the Greater Caribbean and facilitates cooperation and communication among the subregional actors (Asociación de Estados del Caribe (AEC), 2020).

Concluding observations and key lessons

COVID-19 precipitated societies into new ways of living. The economic disruption exposed the profound interdependence woven by contemporary globalisation, and the risks for the CC of heavy dependence on the tourism and travel sector, labour migration and remittances. It showed the vulnerabilities of global production networks and the necessity of diversifying suppliers, preferably exploring possibilities in closer proximity. Caribbean actors should focus more on promoting intraregional trade, deepening economic links with Latin America, and strengthening functional cooperation and regionalism. In terms of addressing external shocks to the fragile small island economies that characterise the region, the pandemic is a 'defining moment for the regional grouping's reorientation' (Bardouille, 2020, p. 2), one which underscores the necessity of regional functional cooperation and foreign policy coordination.

Caribbean governments played key roles in confronting the pandemic and adopting a panoply of public health security strategies. However, future public policies need to go beyond facing the pandemic's immediate impacts. Social and economic reconstruction in the Caribbean demands policies concentrated on reducing income inequality and social marginalisation, creating jobs, diversifying narrow economic bases, integrating digital technologies so as to add real value to education and administrative systems and productive sectors, and adopting sustainable patterns of production and consumption (United Nations Conference on Trade and Development (UNCTAD), 2020).

The responses that have been implemented should push Caribbean governments and regional institutions to further rethink public policies and protocols and build their resilience to cope with future health emergencies and post-emergency scenarios. Statistical collection and data monitoring systems should be strengthened to enable policy-makers and planners to better understand the synergies between health and societal wellbeing in general.

The current global pandemic occurred partly because of human abuse of the natural environment, specifically via the illegal wildlife trade. This also happens in areas of the Caribbean. The pandemic presents an opportunity to rethink our relationship with the environment, particularly in terms of the threats to human life and biodiversity brought about by poor regulation. It is time for the Caribbean, as an environmentally vulnerable and climate-sensitive region, to find comprehensive ways of accounting for and better regulating the impact of human activity on its natural environment. This is particularly important as most CC states will be looking to diversify their economies and reduce their reliance on tourism and commodity exports.

The findings of the paper confirm the need to embrace multidimensional development concretely and pursue human welfare as the central goal of development. Economic growth, while essential, will not automatically bring social development. The latter must be deliberately and strategically pursued. Despite their long-standing advocacy for broader notions of development as policy drivers, Caribbean countries were caught off guard by the crisis. Inadequacies in the region's education, health and social protection systems were laid bare early in the pandemic. Notwithstanding the stellar efforts of governments to mitigate adverse social impacts and prevent systemic collapse, gaps were apparent. The COVID-19 crisis presents an opportunity to re-engineer governance models, reimagine the social contract and explore how to provide a stronger social safety net for the population in general. An ideal people-centred approach should be institutionalised to withstand changes of government, it should balance the needs of people with physical infrastructural development, and social protection should be equitable, inclusive, participatory and bottom up.

Notes

1. There are twelve independent Caribbean member states of the Commonwealth – Antigua and Barbuda, The Bahamas, Barbados, Belize, Dominica, Grenada, Guyana, Jamaica, St Kitts and Nevis, St Lucia, St Vincent and the Grenadines, and Trinidad and Tobago.
2. Resilience is understood here as the policy-induced ability of an economy to withstand or recover from the negative effects of external shocks (Briguglio et al., 2009). We extend this somewhat to discuss social as well as economic resilience.
3. Island geographies lend themselves to measures like border closures and quarantines. Anecdotal evidence suggests that continental CC territories experienced greater challenges

with border security management as infection rates escalated in neighbouring countries. The downside of long-term closure is that CC open economies depend heavily on importation, international tourism and travel, labour migration and remittances, activities which emphasise mobility and an umbilical cord relationship with the global economy. Hemispheric geopolitics have exercised cross-cutting effects on the CC, facilitating cooperation with hemispheric neighbours, but also requiring skilful manoeuvring through the cross-hairs of deteriorating US-China relations and growing hegemonic pressure on actors in the Greater Caribbean.

4. Guyana's exploitation of recently discovered offshore petroleum resources is projected to generate GDP growth of 44.3% in 2020 (ECLAC, 2020b: 8).
5. St Lucia recorded 171 cases and 59 recoveries. It registered its first death on 10 November 2020 and up to the time of writing has had two deaths. St Vincent has recorded 78 cases, Dominica 68 cases, Grenada 32 cases, St Kitts and Nevis 19 cases, all with no deaths.
6. In Belize, about 25% of surveyed households indicated skipping of meals or reduced food intake.
7. Examples of both circumstances include the Jamaican government calling national elections six months before they were constitutionally due, while in St. Kitts and Nevis, elections due by March 2020 were postponed until June due to the challenge of organising the poll during a state of emergency.
8. Anguilla, Belize, Bermuda, Dominican Republic, Guyana, Jamaica, Puerto Rico, St. Kitts and Nevis, St. Vincent and the Grenadines, Suriname, Trinidad and Tobago.
9. Ensuring a peaceful resolution to the political crisis in Guyana assumed great significance for the Caribbean Community, as for the Commonwealth and the Organisation of American States, because of the region's democratic norms, because of the location of the CARICOM headquarters in Guyana and because of Guyana's growing socio-economic significance in the region and the hemisphere (Trotz & Bulkan, 2020; Larocque, 2020).
10. Sources: CARICOM Secretariat; Caribbean Elections; Guyana News and Information; Stabroek News; GECOM; Trinidad Express (2020); St. Kitts-Nevis Observer; RJR/Gleaner; Caribbean Council (2020); Belize Electoral Council (2020); Nation News.BBC; Electoral Commission of Jamaica (2020); Electoral Office Government of St Vincent and the Grenadines (2020)
11. There are many critiques concerning the shortcomings of Guyana's party list quota system. See Hosein & Parpart (2017), and Faieta, McDade and Arias (2019).
12. This is a sensitive issue in CC SIDS with high migration and remittance profiles.
13. Trinidad is the only CC state to have taken the initiative to provide temporary residence and work permits for over 15,000 Venezuelan migrants in July 2019. Its geographical proximity to Venezuela, coupled with the deteriorating humanitarian situation there and the challenges of the pandemic mean that Trinidad is caught between national security concerns and humanitarian considerations (Amnesty International, 2020; Caribbean National Weekly, 2020; United Nations High Commission for Refugees, 2020).

Disclosure statement

No potential conflict of interest was reported by the authors.

References

Allen, P. (2020, August 12). *Trinidad and Tobago expects COVID-19 surge following elections.* Caribbean Business Report. https://caribbeanbusinessreport.com/news/tt-expects-covid-19-surge-following-elections/

Amnesty International. (2020, August 8). *Trinidad and Tobago: Deportation of 165 Venezuelans violates international law.* https://www.amnesty.org/en/countries/americas/trinidad-and-tobago

Asociación de Estados del Caribe (AEC). (2020, July 31). *Declaración de la XXV Reunión Ordinaria del Consejo de Ministros de la Asociación de Estados del Caribe (AEC) sobre el COVID-19, MC/2020/25/Anexo.033.* http://www.acs-aec.org/sites/default/files/mc202025rrannex033es.pdf

Attzs, M. (2020). *Civil society is rebuilding resilience in coronavirus-stricken Caribbean.* Devex. https://www.devex.com/news/opinion-civil-society-is-rebuilding-resilience-in-coronavirus-stricken-caribbean-97415

Baptiste, D. (2020, June 27). *PM Browne on LIAT liquidation: Hundreds will lose their jobs.* LOOP TT. https://www.looptt.com/content/pm-browne-liat-liquidation-hundreds-will-lose-their-jobs-5

Bardouille, N. C. (2020, August 24). *The Coronavirus (COVID-19) and the Caribbean: Economic, governance and political contexts.* SRC Working Paper. Caribbean Studies Association (CSA). https://www.caribbeanstudiesassociation.org/src-working-paper-the-coronavirus-covid-19-and-the-caribbean-economic-governance-and-political-contexts/

Basile, G. (2020). SARS-CoV-2 en América Latina y Caribe: Las tres encrucijadas para el pensamiento crítico en salud. *Ciência & Saúde Coletiva, 25*(9), 3557–3562. https://doi.org/10.1590/1413-81232020259.20952020

Beuermann, D. W., Álvarez, L. G., Hoffmann, B., & Vera Cossio, D. (2020), *COVID-19, The Caribbean crisis.* https://blogs.iadb.org/caribbean-dev-trends/en/covid-19-the-caribbean-crisis/

Bishop, M. L., & Payne, A. (2010, January). *Caribbean regional governance and the sovereignty/statehood problem* CIGI Caribbean Paper No. 8. www.cigionline.org

Briguglio, L., Cordina, G., Farrugia, N., & Vella, S. (2009). Economic vulnerability and resilience: Concepts and measurements'. *Oxford Development Studies, 37*(3), 229–247. https://doi.org/10.1080/13600810903089893

Byron, J. (2014). Developmental regionalism in crisis? Rethinking CARICOM, deepening relations with Latin America. *Caribbean Journal of International Relations and Diplomacy, 2*(4), 23–50. https://journals.sta.uwi.edu/ojs/index.php/iir/article/view/509/431

Byron, J. (2016). Summitry in the Caribbean Community: A Fundamental Feature of Regional Governance. In G. Mace, J.-P. Therien, D. Tussie, & O. Dabene (Eds.), *Summits and regional governance: The Americas in comparative perspective* (pp. 88–105). Routledge.

Caribbean Council. (2020a, April 21). *CARICOM Heads agree to develop common responses to challenges posed by COVID 19.* www.caribbean-council.org/caricom-heads-to-develop-common-responses-to-challenges-posed-by-COVID-19

Caribbean Council. (2020b, May 19). *CARICOM Heads agree to steps required to reopen the regional economy.* www.caribbean-council.org/caricom-heads-agree-to-steps-required-to-reopen-the-regional-economy/

Caribbean Council. (2020c, June 1). *Caribbean Governments taking different approaches on timing to reopen tourism.* www.caribbean-council.org/caribbean-govts-taking-different-approaches-on-timing_to-reopen-tourism/

CARICOM Secretariat. (2020, February 26). *Working Group established to make recommendations for regional response to COVID-19.* www.today.caricom.org/2020/02/26/working-group-to-concretise-recommendations-for-a-regional-response-to-covid-19/

CARPHA. (2020). *COVID-19 background.* https://carpha.org/What-We-Do/Public-Health/Novel-Coronavirus/COVID-19-Background

Casas-Zamora, K. (2020, October 1). *Democracy in a time of crisis.* International Institute for Democracy and Electoral Assistance. www.idea.int/news-media/media/democracy-time-crisis

CNG News. (2020, September 29). *St Lucia Bar association intervenes on COVID-19 Bill.* https://www.caribbeannewsglobal.com/st-lucia-bar-association-intervenes-on-covid-19-bill/

Collins, R. (2008). Strengthening the Caribbean community: A comment on the role of functional cooperation. In K. Hall & M. Chuck-A-Sang (Eds.), *The Caribbean community in transition: Functional cooperation as a catalyst for change* (pp. 3–10). Ian Randle Publishers.

Comisión Económica para América Latina y el Caribe (CEPAL). (2020). *Estudio Económico de América Latina y el Caribe 2020.* Santiago. https://repositorio.cepal.org/bitstream/handle/11362/46070/89/S2000371_es.pdf

Coronavirus Resources Center at John Hopkins University. John Hopkins University. https://coronavirus.jhu.edu/map.html

Dhanpaul, V. (2020). *'Where the money gone?' Mystery or mischief?.* Ministry of Finance, Government of the Republic of Trinidad & Tobago. https://www.finance.gov.tt/wp-content/uploads/2020/09/Vishnu-Dhanpaul-Final-Cash-Flow-January-to-June-Spotlight-on-the-Budget-2021-Final.pdf

Doyle, C., & Patel, P. (2008). Civil society organisations and global health initiatives: Problems of legitimacy. *Social Science & Medicine, 66*(9), 1928–1938. https://doi.org/10.1016/j.socscimed.2007.12.029

Dukharan, M. (2020, March 3). *COVID-19 Caribbean economic impact report.* Marla Dukharan webpage. https://marladukharan.com/wp-content/uploads/2020/03/MD-COVID19-Caribbean-Economic-Impacts.pdf

Economic Commission for Latin America and the Caribbean (ECLAC). (2020a). *Economic survey of Latin America and the Caribbean 2020.* (LC/PUB.2020/12-P).

Economic Commission for Latin America and the Caribbean (ECLAC). (2020b). *The Caribbean outlook: Forging a people-centred approach sustainable development post-COVID-19.* (LC/SES.38/12).

Electoral Commission of Jamaica. (2020). Government of Jamaica. www.ecj.com.jm/elections/election-results/

Electoral Office Government of St Vincent and the Grenadines. (2020) *'Election results 2020'.* www.electoral.gov.vc/electoral.index.php/election/results/

Faieta, J., McDade, S., & Arias, R. (2019, July 26). *Where are the women? A study of women, politics, parliaments and equality in the Commonwealth Caribbean countries.* UNDP Report. https://iknowpolitics.org/sites/default/files/jm_where_are_the_women_caricom.pdf

Flowers, Y. C. (2020). *COVID-19 and education in Belize,* http://tcg.uis.unesco.org/wp-content/uploads/sites/4/2020/05/UIS_COVID_Belize.pdf

GECOM. (2020, August 24). *Gazetted declaration of results of general and regional elections 2020.* Government of Guyana. www.gecom.gy

Girvan, N. (2010). Caribbean community: The elusive quest for economic integration. In F. Alleyne, D. Lewis-Bynoe, & X. Archibald (Eds.), *Growth and development strategies in the Caribbean* (pp. 199–218). Caribbean Development Bank.

Government of Belize Elections and Boundaries Department. (2020) *'Elections results November 12 2020'* Government of Belize. www.elections.gov.bz

Government of the Republic of Trinidad & Tobago. (2020). *Stability, strength, growth.* Ministry of Finance. https://www.finance.gov.tt/publications/national-budget/review-of-the-economy/

Healthy Caribbean Coalition. (2020, March 27). *Open letter to CARICOM Heads of state and government about NCDs and COVID-19.* https://www.healthycaribbean.org/hcc-open-letter-to-caricom-heads-of-state-and-government-about-ncds-and-covid-19/

Hosein, G., & Parpart, J. (eds). (2017). *Negotiating gender policy and politics in the Caribbean: Feminist strategies, masculinist resistance and transformational possibilities.* Rowman and Littlefield.

Hunte, S., Pierre, K., St. Rose, R., & Simeon, D. (2020). Health systems' resilience: COVID-19 response in Trinidad and Tobago. *American Journal of Tropical Medicine & Hygiene, 103*(2), 590–592. https://doi.org/10.4269/ajtmh.20-0561

Imbert, C. (2020). *Budget 2021 core data presented by The Minister of finance on Sep 28, 2020 at the spotlight on the budget and economy.* Ministry of Finance, Government of the Republic of Trinidad & Tobago. Powerpoint presentation. https://www.finance.gov.tt/wp-content/uploads/2020/09/Honourable-Colm-Imbert-Minister-of-Finance-Spotlight-on-the-Budget-2021-Presentation.pdf

IMF. (2020) *Policy tracker.* https://www.imf.org/en/Topics/imf-and-covid19/Policy-Responses-to-COVID-19#A

Interamerican Development Bank (IADB). (2020, May 15). *CARPHA receiving additional support to fight COVID-19.* https://www.iadb.org/en/news/carpha-receiving-additional-support-fight-covid-19

International IDEA. (2020, September 30). *Going against the trend: elections with increased voter turnout during the COVID-19 pandemic.* www.idea.int/news-medi/news/going-against-trend-elections-increased-voter-turnout-during-covid-19-pandemic

Knight, A., & Reddy Srikanth, R. (2020). Caribbean response to COVID-19: A regional approach to pandemic preparedness and resilience. *The Round Table, 109*(4), 464–465. https://doi.org/10.1080/00358533.2020.1790759

Larocque, I. (2020, July 3). CARICOM. www.caricom.org.remarks-by-caricom-secretary-general-ambassador-irwin-larocque-to-the-20th-special-meeting-of-caricom-heads-of-government/

LoopNews. (2020, May 15). *NGO: Environment must be part of 'roadmap to recovery', post-COVID -19.* Loop News - Trend Media. https://www.looptt.com/content/ngo-environment-must-be-part-roadmap-recovery-post-covid-19

McDonald, S. (2020, January 24). A busy year in the Caribbean: Elections. www.csis.org/analysis/busy-year-caribbean-elections/

McKenzie, N. (2020, April 17). *COVID-19 crisis has exposed societal gaps.* Eyewitness News. https://ewnews.com/covid-19-crisis-has-exposed-societal-gaps

Mera, M. (2020). Social and economic impact of the COVID-19 and policy options in Jamaica UNDP Latin America and the Caribbean.

Ministerio de Relaciones Exteriores de la República de Cuba (MINREX). (2020 July 21). *Actualización del mapa infográfico. Brigadas médicas cubanas 'Henry Reeve' para enfrentar la pandemia provocada por la Covid-19.* CubaMINREX. http://www.minrex.gob.cu/es/mapa-info grafico-brigadas-medicas-cubanas-henry-reeve-en-el-enfrentamiento-la-covic19-en-el-mundo

Mooney, H., & Zegorra, M. A. (2020, June 30). *IADB report extreme outlier: The pandemic's unexpected shock to tourism.* Inter-American Development Bank. https://doi.org/10.18235/0002470

Mottley, M. (2020 July 3). *Remarks by the Honourable Mia Amor Mottley prime minister of Barbados as outgoing chair of CARICOM during the 20th special meeting of CARICOM Heads.* CARICOM. www.caricom.org/remarks-by-the-hon-mia-amor-mottley-prime-minister-of-barbados-as-outgoing-chair-of-caricom-during-the-20th-special-meeting-of-caricom-heads

Nanton, S. (2020, October 1). *Caribbean Airlines to make temporary cuts in staff, salaries.* Trinidad & Tobago Guardian. https://www.guardian.co.tt/news/caribbean-airlines-to-make-temporary-cuts-in-staff-salaries-6.2.1224975.18120c7bdc#:~:text=It%20announced%20that%20in%20the,for%20those%20on%20higher%20remuneration.%E2%80%9D

OECS Commission. (2020a). *COVID-19 and beyond: Impact assessments and responses.* https://oecs.org

OECS Commission. (2020b). *OECS education sector response and recovery strategy to COVID-19.* OECS. https://www.oecs.org/our-work/knowledge/library/oecs-education-sector-response-strategy-to-covid-19/viewdocument/2115

PAHO and WHO. (2017), *The role of civil society and community in health policy-making,* https://www.paho.org/salud-en-las-americas-2017/?p=71

Ram, J. (2020). *COVID-19 policy responses for the Caribbean.*

Robinson, C. (2020, August 23). *Election spike – Jamaica to see surge in Covid-19 cases in the wake of polls, warns medic.* The Gleaner Jamaica. www.jamaica-gleaner.com/article.lead-stories /20200823/election-spike-jamaica-see-surge-covid-19-cases-wake-poll-warns-medic

Rodriguez, L. (2020, April 28). *Powerful women leaders from around the world are working together to fight COVID-19.* Global Citizen. https://www.globalcitizen.org/en/content/un-rise-for-all-covid -19-recovery-initiative/

Simoes, A., & Hidalgo, C. (2011). *The economic complexity observatory: An analytical tool for understanding the dynamics of economic development. Paper presented at the Workshops at the Twenty-Fifth AAAI Conference on Artificial Intelligence,* San Francisco, CA.

Smith, J., Buse, K., & Gordon, C. (2016). Civil society: The catalyst for ensuring health in the age of sustainable development. *Globalization and Health*, *12*(40), 1–6. https://doi.org/10.1186/s12992-016-0178

Stabroek News. (2020a, August 12). *Trinidad: Doctor fears spike in Covid-19 cases following election.* https://www.stabroeknews.com/2020/08/12/news/regional/trinidad/trinidad-doctor-fears-spike-in-covid-19-cases-following-election/

Stabroek News. (2020b, September 16). *CARICOM agrees to 'travel bubble'.* https://www.stabroeknews.com/2020/09/16/news/guyana/caricom-agrees-travel-bubble/

Storeng, K. T., & Puyvalle, A. (2018). Civil society participation in global public private partnerships for health. *Health Policy and Planning*, *1–9*(8), 928–936. https://doi.org/10.1093/heapol/czy070

Sunday Express. (2020, August 4). *PNM leads by 5%.* https://trinidadexpress.com/elections/2020/politics/pnm-leads-by-5-pt-1/article_2d8d9ada-d45a-11ea-bl3/

Sutton, P. (2007). Democracy and good governance in small states. In E. Kisanga & S. J. Danchie (Eds.), *Commonwealth small states: Issues and Prospects* (pp. 201–217). Commonwealth Secretariat/Commonwealth Parliamentary Association.

Taitt, R. (2020 August 8). *Responses were too late: Rowley blames lack of finance for no election observers in Trinidad and Tobago.* Jamaica Observer. www.trinidadexpress.com/elections/2020/politics/responses-were-too-late/article_b692154ca-elba-llea-8e37-bfdcc7898d8f.html

The Economist. (2020, August 20). The pandemic's indirect hit on the Caribbean. *The Economist.* https://www.economist.com/the-americas/2020/08/20/the-pandemics-indirect-hit-on-the-caribbean

The UWI St Augustine. (2020, April 21). *Addressing gender-based violence is essential to COVID-19 response and recovery.* News release. https://sta.uwi.edu/news/releases/release.asp?id=1473

Thompson, C. (2020, September 16). *The 2020 General election and the future of the PNP.* Jamaica Observer. www.jamaicaobserver.com/opinion/the-2020-general-election-and-the-future-of-the-pnp_202658?profile=1096

Trotz, A., & Bulkan, A. (2020, June 30). *Guyana's political tragedy.* Stabroek News. https://www.stabroeknews.com/2020/06/30/features/in-the-diaspora/guyanas-political-tragedy/

UNAIDS. (2020, May 18). *COVID-19 community support for Trinidadians on the margins.* https://www.unaids.org/en/resources/presscentre/featurestories/2020/may/20200518_trinidad-and-tobago

UNESCO. (2020). *Teacher development for online and blended learning to ensure quality education during COVID-19 in Jamaica.* https://en.unesco.org/news/teacher-development-online-and-blended-learning-ensure-quality-education-during-covid-19

UNICEF (2020). *Call to action to governments to utilize comprehensive social protection to respond to COVID 19UNICEF (2020). 5 ways COVID-19 is affecting children in Belize and how UNICEF is helping.* https://www.unicef.org/belize/stories/5-ways-covid-19-affecting-children-belize

UNICEF and UN Women Eastern Caribbean. (2020a), *Antigua and Barbuda COVID-19 heat report human and economic assessment of impact.* https://www.bb.undp.org/content/barbados/en/home/library/undp_publications/human-and-economic-assessment-of-impact-antigua-and-barbuda.html

United Nations Conference on Trade and Development (UNCTAD). (2020). *Trade and development report 2020. from global pandemic to prosperity for all: Avoiding another lost decade.* https://unctad.org/en/PublicationsLibrary/tdr2020_en.pdf

United Nations Economic Commission for Latin America and the Caribbean (ECLAC). (2020, April 21). *Measuring the impact of COVID-19 with a view to reactivation. Special report COVID-19.* N. 2. https://repositorio.cepal.org/bitstream/handle/11362/45477/6/S2000285_en.pdf

United Nations High Commission for Refugees. (2020, June 2). *R4V guidance note: Mitigation of risks of eviction for refugees and migrants from Venezuela.* https://data2.unhcr.org/es/documents/details/77042

USAID and UNESCO. (2020), *The socio-economic impact of COVID-19 on children and young people in the Eastern Caribbean area*. UNICEF. https://www.unicef.org/easterncaribbean/media/1956/file/Socio-economic%20Impact.pdf

Wilkinson, E. (2020, May 18). *COVID-19: A lesson in leadership from the Caribbean*. ODI. https://www.odi.org/blogs/16959-covid-19-lesson-leadership-caribbean

Wyss, J. (2020, September 3). *Jamaica holds election with success story shattered by virus*. Bloomberg Quint. https://www.bloombergquint.com/onweb/jamaica-holds-elections-with-success-story-shattered-by-covid-19

Australia and New Zealand: the pandemic Down Under

Derek McDougall

ABSTRACT

Australia and New Zealand have done relatively well in international terms in combating COVID-19, aided by their geographical isolation and political leadership. Overall, they have pursued strategies of assertive suppression in relation to the virus, varying to some extent between 'softer' and 'harder' versions, as among the federal government in Australia, the various Australian states and territories, and New Zealand. Economically both countries have experienced a recession, New Zealand more so than Australia. Governments in both countries have pursued Keynesian policies, acting decisively to provide wage support and assist businesses. The assumption is that these policies will provide the necessary stimulus to prevent economic collapse and to enhance the prospects for subsequent economic recovery. Internationally the relative success of Australia and New Zealand in responding to COVID enhances their ability to influence the post-COVID world. While Australia as the larger country is better positioned in this respect, New Zealand also has considerable 'soft power'.

Introduction

With the onset of COVID-19 in Wuhan, China, in December 2019, most countries of the world have been affected, although to varying degrees. Australia and New Zealand are no exception. This article examines how the two countries have responded to the pandemic, focusing on public health and economic issues, before discussing the changed geopolitical circumstances for the governments in Canberra and Wellington. Initially, there is an overview of the political arrangements underpinning the Australian and New Zealand responses. In relation to the public health and economic dimensions, we ask how well the various governments have done with their responses. Looking to the future, there is the question of whether the pandemic will lead to major changes in Australia and New Zealand; geopolitically too, we ask whether the two countries are likely to be advantaged or disadvantaged by the circumstances that are unfolding as a result of the pandemic.

Internationally Australia and New Zealand have done relatively well in responding to the pandemic, indicating effective political leadership. Both countries responded early, although there have been some differences of emphasis both within Australia and between Australia and New Zealand in relation to both health and economic issues. Given that so many other countries have done so much worse, both Australia and New Zealand are well positioned to take advantage of changed economic and strategic circumstances post-pandemic. This is not to say, of course, that Australia and New Zealand would not have been better off without the pandemic in absolute terms. It is merely a statement about relativities and does not belittle the immense challenges that both countries face in returning to 'normal'.

Background

While the pandemic began in China at the end of 2019, it was not until February 2020 that Australia and New Zealand began to act.

In examining the responses to the pandemic, the relevant political arrangements in Australia and New Zealand need to be noted. Australia is a federal system, with responsibilities for health divided between the federal government and the states. The federal government has superior financial power, providing much of the funding for hospitals and the national health insurance scheme (Medicare), as well as monitoring quality and safety and contributing substantially to the funding of aged care; the states run the public hospitals, and have day-to-day responsibilities for public health. In relation to economic matters, the federal government is responsible for overall national economic management, and also funds social welfare through such means as unemployment benefits and various pension schemes; the states promote economic activity within their own jurisdictions, as well as being major employers (sometimes through outsourcing) in areas such as education, health, public transport and infrastructure construction. In the case of New Zealand, it has a unitary system whereby the functions that are divided in Australia are the responsibility of the one national government. New Zealand also has a smaller population than does Australia: just over five million as compared to 25.5 million.

In the Australian case the response to the pandemic has been managed through the institution of a National Cabinet (from 13 March 2020), involving the prime minister, the six state premiers, and the two chief ministers from territories (Northern Territory, Australian Capital Territory). The National Cabinet represents an evolution of the federal-state cooperation embodied in the Council of Australian Governments (COAG); on 29 May 2020 Prime Minister Scott Morrison announced that a National Federation Reform Council (NFRC), centred on National Cabinet, would replace COAG. In terms of party identification, the current federal government is based on the centre-right Liberal-National Coalition; three of the states have governments of the same persuasion (New South Wales (Coalition), South Australia (Liberal), Tasmania (Liberal), with the remaining three having Labor (centre-left) governments (Queensland, Victoria, Western Australia). The advice coming from chief medical/health officers at both federal and state levels has been very important in determining the response to COVID-19; the formal body for the federal and state chief medical/health officers is the Australian Health Protection Principal Committee (AHPPC). It should be noted that the National Cabinet is essentially a coordinating body; the federal government and the states retain their respective responsibilities as outlined above, meaning that divergences can occur between the federal and state governments, and among the states themselves.

With New Zealand's unitary government, normal cabinet government has prevailed under the leadership of Prime Minister Jacinda Ardern (Labour), with the health minister and chief medical officer also being key figures. Australia and New Zealand have cooperated with their responses to the pandemic, with Ardern joining a meeting of the National Cabinet in Australia on 5 May 2020.

In responding to the pandemic, the major challenge has been to strike a balance between what is best for public health (described below) and the need to limit damage to the economy. While initially there was a high level of cooperation among the various jurisdictions involved, over time there have been differences, mainly focusing on arguments about what the right balance should be.

The public health response

In the domain of public health, various strategies have been proposed and attempted. At one end of the spectrum there is a strategy of doing little, either because of a belief that COVID-19 is of minimal significance (the position of President Jair Bolsonaro in Brazil) or because of the view that allowing the virus to spread encourages the development of 'herd immunity' (for example, Sweden), thus protecting most people in the long term. The negative side of this strategy is that the number of cases can explode, putting pressure on hospital facilities and ensuring that many more people die than would otherwise be the case. At the other end of the spectrum there is the elimination strategy whereby an attempt is made to locate and isolate all cases of COVID-19 within a particular jurisdiction, ensuring also that no new cases arrive from outside that setting; this approach suits situations that are relatively isolated from the outside world (or can be), such as Taiwan and Iceland. Between these two strategies other possibilities include mitigation and suppression. Mitigation entails minimal measures to contain the virus, acting to deal with the worst impacts, but largely relying on people to exercise common sense in relation to distancing and other measures that might reduce the spread of the virus. Suppression offers a range of possibilities in terms of the intensity of the measures to be implemented. The aim is to reduce the spread of the virus to such a point that normal life can be resumed, but without assuming that it can ever be implemented completely.

These different strategies also allow for some time elapsing before a vaccine to combat coronavirus becomes widely available (and even then, might not offer complete protection).

Given the different possible strategies, Australia (meaning the federal government, the states and the territories) opted for an assertive form of suppression, varying to some extent among the different jurisdictions; New Zealand's strategy aimed for a 'hard' version of suppression, something close to elimination. Both countries sought to minimise the economic impact. New Zealand concluded that a period with the highest level of restrictions would enable the virus to be eliminated or virtually so; the economic pain would be considerable in the short term, but that pain was preferable to having a long drawn out period of economic hardship with no guarantee that the virus would disappear. In the Australian case the arguments for a suppression strategy prevailed, but there were variations on the issue of how assertive that strategy should be; it was a question of determining the best balance between the health and economic costs. The federal government generally preferred a 'softer' strategy; states such as Western Australia and Tasmania were more 'hard line'. Both Australia and New Zealand were in a position where they could isolate themselves to a large extent from the outside world. Within Australia it was also possible for states to isolate themselves from each other, with Queensland, South Australia, Tasmania and Western Australia doing this to varying degrees (and also New South Wales in relation to Victoria from August to November 2020).

Australia

The major steps in the unfolding of the pandemic strategy in Australia (allowing for some differences among the states) can be seen by referring to key dates (based on Ting & Palmer, 2020).

In Australia, the pandemic moved to the top of the public agenda with increasing awareness of COVID-19 spreading from China during January 2020. On 31 January, the World Health Organization (WHO) declared a 'public health emergency of international concern'; on 11 March it declared an official pandemic. Australia blocked passenger arrivals from China beginning 1 February. However more drastic measures were yet to come.

Indicative in this respect was a statement by Morrison on 27 February that a pandemic was anticipated, with emergency response plans under consideration. The ban on passengers from China was extended to include arrivals from Iran (29 February) and South Korea (5 March). On 13 March, the prime minister announced a ban on non-essential outdoor gatherings over 500 people from 16 March; people arriving from overseas would be required to self-isolate for 14 days; Australians were urged not to travel overseas. From 18 March non-essential indoor gatherings of over 100 people were banned; Australians overseas were advised to return home. From this latter date a federal biosecurity emergency took effect under the Biosecurity Act of 2015.

From 19 March only citizens and residents could enter Australia. This was also the date when the *Ruby Princess*, a cruise ship, disembarked passengers in Sydney; a failure in health checks led to a surge in COVID-19 cases (663 cases and 28 deaths were linked to the ship) (Hair, 2020). Travel restrictions affecting specific states began on 20 March with a ban on non-essential travel to Tasmania.

From 24 March people were advised to work from home where possible; non-essential businesses were to close from 25 March.[1] Australians were now barred from travelling overseas. The Northern Territory, Queensland, South Australia and Western Australia instituted border controls of various kinds; Western Australia closed its borders from 5 April. From 29 March the limit for indoor and outdoor gatherings was set at two people in most cases; there was also compulsory hotel quarantine for 14 days for Australians entering the country.

With international transmission of COVID-19 seemingly under control because of entry for non-Australian citizens (apart from permanent residents) largely barred, there was an easing of the pandemic restrictions. The changes varied depending on the state or territory. The Northern Territory began to lift restrictions during May, with life relatively normal from 5 June (some restrictions on travel into the territory remained). Other jurisdictions moved more slowly, with travel restrictions remaining in the four smaller states, but generally some easing of restrictions within states (life in Western Australia, for example, became relatively normal).

A major setback to the recovery was a worrying rise in the number of cases in Victoria from mid-June, leading to a second wave that made Victoria the state most affected by COVID. The problem appeared to be a failure in the system of quarantining international arrivals in hotels and in the arrangements for contact tracing; proper infectious disease control practices were not implemented in the quarantine hotels (security being outsourced to private security firms), and contact tracing and isolating of the COVID cases were ineffective (90% of the cases in Victoria's second wave arose from one 'superspreader' family).[2] The Victorian government set up a judicial inquiry to investigate the matter, subsequently recommending much clearer governance arrangements for quarantine and a stricter regime of infection prevention and control (Victoria, COVID-19 Hotel Quarantine Inquiry, 2020).

In response to the emerging second wave the Victorian government moved back to more stringent restrictions, increasing these to Stage 4 for Melbourne (but not regional Victoria) on 2 August (to last until 13 September). On 6 September Premier Daniel Andrews announced a 'road map' for Victoria, distinguishing between Melbourne and regional areas, but essentially extending the Stage 4 lockdown beyond 13 September; restrictions would be eased gradually subject to targets being met (number of cases), with the aim of achieving a COVID-normal Christmas.

By this stage there was considerable criticism of Victoria's strategy, the critics essentially arguing that Andrews was being ultra-cautious, as well as claiming that he had been ineffective in dealing with lapses in the hotel quarantine system and the weaknesses of contact tracing. Increasingly loud criticism came from the federal government (concerned about the impact on the economy), business interests and some epidemiologists and other doctors (for example, A Doctors' Open Letter to Dan Andrews, 2020; see also Colebatch, 2020). Articles in *Quadrant* reflected a more strongly stated right wing and libertarian critique, with titles such as 'East Germany on the Yarra' and 'Why the Left Loves the Lockdown'; Victoria became 'Danistan' or 'Sicktoria'; the pandemic became the 'Dandemic'. Victorian Liberal MP Tim Smith, known for his colourful language, declared that the state was 'governed by a bunch of totalitarian leftwing nutters who are going to destroy Victoria' (Alcorn, 2020).

By late October there had been a huge improvement in the situation in Victoria: on 27 October, there were 38 active cases in metropolitan Melbourne (average of 2.7 new cases per day over the previous 14 days); for regional Victoria, there were no cases, with an average of zero over the previous 14 days. By early November Victoria had achieved virtual elimination; as of 15 December, there had been no new cases through community transmission for 46 days (but seven internationally acquired cases with people in hotel quarantine) (Victoria, Department of Health and Human Services, 2020). This rapid improvement enabled an acceleration of Victoria's previously planned 'road map', with some restrictions such as density limits for venues, masking in certain contexts, and requirements for many people to work from home, but generally a much more normal life.

Since COVID-19 disproportionately affects older people, one of the issues has been the situation in aged care homes. The emergence of COVID-19 in an aged care home can lead to its rapid spread within that home. In the earlier period of the pandemic there was a major problem at Newmarch House (under Anglicare, an agency of the Anglican Church) in western Sydney, with 37 cases among residents, 34 among staff, and 17 COVID-attributed deaths among residents in the April-June period (Gilbert & Lilly, 2020, p. 8). With the resurgence of the pandemic in Melbourne from June there were numerous aged care homes affected, one of the worst being St Basil's Homes for the Aged, a facility under the auspices of the Greek Orthodox Church in the northern suburb of Fawkner, with 183 cases and 44 deaths (as of 12 September) (Michie, 2020). Aged care in Australia is predominantly the province of the federal government as the main source of financial support for the system; providers can be businesses or community-based organisations. The federal government had appointed a royal commission to enquire into aged care in Australia (established October 2018; with a final report due, November 2021; in October 2020 the commission issued a report on COVID-19 and aged care); the pandemic has highlighted issues relating to this sector, such as the relationship between homes and hospitals in the event of a pandemic, and the use of contract staff who might work in a number of homes (thus facilitating transmission). The commission pointed out that while a high proportion of Australian deaths from COVID were in aged care (74%, as of 19 September 2020, high by international standards, the mortality rate as a proportion of aged care residents was low (0.25%; for Canada it is 1.5%, and for the United Kingdom it is 5.3%) (Australia, Royal Commission into Aged Care Quality and Safety, 2020, p. 8).

On 19 August 2020 Prime Minister Morrison announced that the federal government had signed an agreement to use a COVID-19 vaccine being developed at the University of Oxford, with commercial aspects under the auspices of AstraZeneca, a British pharmaceutical company. Subsequently there were also agreements with Novovax and Pfizer/BioNTech; Australia also participated in the COVAX Facility to provide options for purchasing other vaccines, as well as assisting developing countries to obtain access to vaccines; in Australia itself the government funded vaccine research at the University of Queensland, but this research did not proceed past the first phase of clinical trials (Australian Government, Department of Health, 2020b, 11 December). Greg Hunt (federal health minister) optimistically predicted in September 2020 that a vaccine would be available to Australians in the first half of 2021, with the first doses possibly as early as late January 2021 (The Morning Show, 2020). Given the beginning of a vaccine rollout in the United Kingdom from early December 2020, Hunt's prediction could well be right.

Overall Australia's public health strategy of assertive suppression achieved a high level of success ahead of the second wave that developed in Victoria from July, and still ranked highly even with that development (Australia ranked 151st out of 215 countries, based on total cases in relation to size of population, Worldometer, 16 December 2020). Table 1 provides statistics on COVID-19 cases (total and active) and deaths in the various Australian states and territories as of mid-December 2020, as well as figures for Australia as a whole. Early in the pandemic there was some variation in approach among the governments involved, but a general image of cooperation. The second

Table 1. COVID-19 Statistics for Australia, 15 December 2020 (figures in brackets indicate percentage of population).

	Total cases	Active cases	Deaths
Victoria	20,351 (0.0304)	7	820 (0.0012)
New South Wales	4,650 (0.0057)	8	53 (0.0006)
Queensland	1228 (0.0024)	17	6 (0.0001)
Western Australia	838 (0.0032)	8	9 (0.0003)
South Australia	563 (0.0032)	1	4 (0.0002)
Tasmania	234 (0.0043)	4	13 (0.0024)
Australian Capital Territory	117 (0.0027)	0	3 (0.0007)
Northern Territory	66 (00.26)	0	0
Australia	28,047 (0.011)	47 (46 international, one under investigation)	908 (0.0004)

Source: Australian Government, Department of Health, 2020a, 16 December, with links to state health departments; per capita figures calculated from population figures according to Australian Bureau of Statistics (2020c, 24 September). The discrepancy between the Australian total for active cases and the figures for states and territories is due to the dynamic nature of the statistics.

wave in Victoria, however, tested the cooperation that had been achieved, with the federal government becoming increasingly critical of the Victorian government. There were also some tensions among the states; understandably states such as Western Australia, where the virus was virtually eliminated, were inclined to isolate themselves from other states. Australia took advantage of its geographical location to isolate itself to a high degree from contact with the outside world; similarly, some states within Australia isolated themselves from other states.

Indicative of the need to avoid complacency in relation to COVID-19, a new outbreak began in Sydney's northern beach suburbs in mid-December 2020, initially through international transmission. Whether this would become a significant 'second wave' remained to be seen. New South Wales began imposing restrictions in the affected suburbs, and then in greater Sydney and adjacent areas; other states limited the movement of people from Sydney and (in the case of Western Australia) from the whole of New South Wales.

New Zealand

Although Australia opted for an assertive suppression strategy rather than elimination (but still achieving a large measure of elimination), its trans-Tasman neighbour decided to opt for an even stronger version of suppression (verging on elimination). The thinking was that a harder lockdown would put the country in a position to control, if not eliminate the virus; less assertive suppression (Australia overall being marginally less assertive, for example) would take longer and not necessarily be effective, thus prolonging the pain. This strategy proved to be effective in the short term; in August, however, some new cases emerged, leading to a suppression strategy that aimed to be strong but flexible according to the specific circumstances where outbreaks might occur.

Paralleling Australia, but with more ambitious goals, New Zealand's public health response began on 3 February with the imposition of restrictions on foreign citizens entering New Zealand from China; those who could enter would need to go into self-isolation (dates from Strongman, 2020). On 28 February there was the first reported case of COVID-19, the person in question entering the country from Iran. From 14 March anyone able to enter New Zealand would be required to self-isolate, apart from those coming from the Pacific. By 19 March there were 28 COVID cases in New Zealand; the government announced the closure of borders except for New Zealand citizens and permanent residents. A level 2 approach moved to level 3 on 23 March, and level 4 on 25 March (New Zealand used 'level' rather than 'stage'). All non-essential businesses were to close, as were schools and other educational institutions.

New Zealand's 'hard' suppression strategy proved relatively effective, at least in the short term (Baker et al., 2020). On 27 April the country ended level 4 restrictions, moving to level 3 on the following day: the highest level of restrictions had lasted for little more than a month. By 8 June there were no more active COVID cases, and New Zealand moved to level 1, allowing businesses and educational institutions to operate normally, and with no limits on the number of people at a gathering; restrictions on international arrivals and departures remained. By 28 May the total number of recorded cases stood at 1504 (including recoveries), with 22 deaths; as of 8 June, there were no active COVID cases.

Some new cases arose in June (totalling nine active cases on 22 June 2022 on 29 June, and 25 on 12 July) as a result of some people arriving from overseas. A new phase arose on 11 August

Table 2. COVID-19 statistics for New Zealand, 16 December 2020 (figures in brackets indicate percentage of population).

Confirmed and probable cases	2100 (0.0041)
Active cases	43 (all international)
Deaths	25 (0.0005)

Source: New Zealand, Ministry of Health, 2020. Per capita figures calculated from population figures from StatsNZ (2020b).

with the discovery of four cases in a family in Auckland, presumed to be through community transmission rather than international transmission. The following day Auckland moved to level 3 restrictions, with the rest of New Zealand being placed on level 2. By 27 August there were 126 active cases in New Zealand, many linked to the Auckland cluster, but including 11 international transmissions. The Auckland cluster centred on an illicit gathering at the Mt Roskill Evangelical Fellowship; Pacific islanders (particularly from the Cook Islands) were predominant.

In the context of the strong suppression strategy, the peak for active cases was 97 on 13 September, moving to 40 by 5 October (six through community transmission, 34 through international transmission). Except for Auckland, the country moved to level 1 on 21 September (Auckland following on 8 October).

While earlier on it appeared that New Zealand had virtually achieved elimination, with hindsight this conclusion was premature. Nevertheless, New Zealand's numbers overall were very low, a situation aided by the country's geographical isolation and strong leadership under a unitary government. (New Zealand ranked 180th out of 215 countries, based on total cases relative to population, Worldometer, 16 December 2020). Table 2 provides statistics on COVID-19 cases (total and active) and deaths in New Zealand as of mid-December 2020; reference to Table 1 provides a comparison with Australia.

The economic response

While the number of cases of COVID-19 might have been small in both Australia and New Zealand, the major concern has been about the negative economic impact of the health measures adopted.

The major economic impact arises from the fact that so many businesses and other services are closed or reduced in scale to limit the human interaction that facilitates the spread of the virus. This is most obvious in areas such as hospitality and tourism, but closures and reduction in scale can extend to many other sectors. Stage 4 restrictions usually mean that people are confined to home, except for exercise and outside excursions relating to shopping for groceries, medical attention and 'caring'. Stage 3 restrictions cover the same ground but allow more businesses to remain open (for example, take away food), subject to distancing. Masks might be made mandatory with either level of restrictions.

Australia

With Stage 3 restrictions coming into force in the various jurisdictions in Australia during March, the effect was to force the closure or partial closure of businesses in sectors such as hospitality and tourism. Workers were required to work from home if that were possible, although public transport continued to operate, as did most of the construction industry. Widespread job losses were reflected in the jump in unemployment; according to the Australian Bureau of Statistics the unemployment rate in June 2020 was 7.4%, 2.2% higher than in June 2019 (note that these figures disguise the 'real' level of unemployment because they are based on the number of people registered as seeking work, thus obscuring the fact that many job seekers would not register). Underemployment (allowing for people who would prefer to work more hours) was 11.7% in June 2020, an increase of 3.5% since June 2019 (Australian Bureau of Statistics, 2020b, 16 July).

To assist individuals in affected businesses the federal government instituted a JobKeeper payment of A$1500 per fortnight for employees in businesses adversely affected by the pandemic; originally due to last until September, this scheme was subsequently extended to March 2021 but with lower payments. Individuals could access their superannuation for a sum of up to A$10,000 in the 2019–2020 financial year and a further A$10,000 in the 2020–2021 financial year if they could establish economic hardship (applicants were not checked initially although there were promises that eligibility would be assessed by the Australian Taxation Office). Improved payments for the unemployed were available through the JobSeeker programme, with a coronavirus supplement of A$550 per fortnight until September (then extended to the end of the year on the basis of A$250 per fortnight) added to the basic fortnightly payment of A$565.70 (single, no children). There were two coronavirus payments of A$750 made to various kinds of pensioners and other concession card holders. Apart from payments to individuals, there was support for business through such means as assisting with short term cash flow problems and improved access to loans. The aim of these various schemes was to prevent the Australian economy from sliding too far into recession and indeed depression.

Figures on the Australian economy indicated a decline of 7.0% in Gross Domestic Product in the June quarter, the worst on record (Australian Bureau of Statistics, 2020a, 2 September). The situation appeared comparable to the post-1929 Great Depression. However, such a judgement would have been premature: subsequent figures for the September quarter showed some recovery with a growth of 3.3% (Australian Bureau of Statistics, 2020d, 2 December).

To finance its schemes to prop up the economy, the federal government borrowed on a massive scale. The federal budget of 6 October 2020 indicated a deficit of A$213.7 billion for 2020–2021 or 11.0% of GDP, with overall economic response and support amounting to A$507 billion (Australian Government, 2020). Net debt for the federal government in 2020–2021 totalled A$703.2billion (36.1% of GDP); for 2023–2024 the estimate was A$966.2 billion (43.8% of GDP) (Australian Government, 2020). State governments similarly committed themselves to higher levels of spending but were less well-resourced than the federal government; the Victorian government, for example, recorded a deficit of A $6.5 billion for the 2019–2020 financial year (the latter part being affected by COVID), with net debt increasing by A$18.4 billion to A$44 billion (Rollason & Staff, 2020). Servicing and reducing the debt for both the federal and state governments would be a long-term exercise, aided by record low interest rates.

A very significant impact of the pandemic was in relation to immigration. Australia as a high immigration country relied on immigrants as a means of expanding the population and stimulating the economy. Travel restrictions meant that immigration would be much less a feature of Australian life. Based on 2018–2019 when net migration was almost 240,000, the expected fall in 2019–2020 was 30% and for 2020–2021 85% (Truu, 2020). A report by Deloitte Access Economics in October 2020 stated that Australia's population growth in 2021 would be 600,000 less than previously predicted (Remeikis, 2020).

Travel restrictions also meant a very severe impact on aviation. This applied both internationally and in relation to restrictions within Australia. Federal support for aviation amounted to A$715 million. Qantas, the main international and domestic carrier, had very limited domestic services and ceased international flights (apart from 'rescue' flights arranged with the government to bring Australians home). Qantas laid off 6000 workers in June, with a further 2500 job losses likely after further announcements in August; it posted a A$2 billion annual loss in August. Virgin Australia, the second most important airline, went into voluntary administration in April 2020 with debts of A$6.8 billion; it was sold in September 2020 to US private equity firm Bain Capital for A$3.5 billion. About 3000 Virgin staff (one third of the workforce) lost their jobs.

Another aspect of Australian life that was affected by the pandemic was education. Depending on the state, schools were closed for long periods; in Victoria, the state with schools closed for the longest period, students returned on a longer-term basis in October. In higher education, campuses were closed. Most significantly it became impossible for international students to enter Australia, thus adversely affecting university budgets, and leading to large scale staff redundancies. International education was ranked as Australia's third most important export industry (after iron ore and coal).

In childcare there is significant involvement by private providers, with federal government assistance of various kinds available to parents. With the onset of COVID many parents withdrew their children, threatening the collapse of the sector. To forestall this possibility the federal government provided direct financial support for childcare centres in the period from April to mid-July on condition that there was no charge for places. Thereafter there was a return to more normal arrangements, but with different kinds of federal support available depending on the restrictions applying in a particular state.

New Zealand

Compared with Australia, the economic impact of COVID in New Zealand has been more severe. In the June quarter (2020), the contraction in GDP was 12.2% (Roy, 2020), nearly twice that experienced in Australia. The unemployment rate in the June quarter actually fell from 4.2% to 4.0% (however this measure requires people to be actively seeking work); more accurately the underutilisation rate (measuring the extent to which people who would normally be part of the labour force were unemployed) rose from 10.4 to 12.0%, with hours worked falling by 10.0% (both records) (StatsNZ, 2020a).

As in Australia, New Zealand instituted wage subsidies to assist the unemployed, and gave support to business. On 17 March 2020 Grant Robertson, the Minister for Finance, announced a COVID-19 Economic Response Package worth NZ$12.1 billion or 4.0% of GDP, claimed to be one of the most generous commitments in the world on a per capita basis. Included in the total were NZ$5.1 billion for wage subsidies, NZ$2.8 billion in income support for the most vulnerable, and NZ$2.8 billion in business tax changes (to assist cash flow) (Robertson, 2020). In the May 2020 Budget there was a NZ$50 billion COVID Response and Recovery Fund (CRRF), a set of measures designed to stimulate the economy and protect society through increased government spending on a range of services. At the time of the May Budget, the government's COVID-related spending amounted to 13% of GDP (11% in Australia); the government's net debt would increase from 20% of GDP to over 55% (Eaqub, 2020).

On specific matters, the closure of borders meant very restricted aviation services, and immigration effectively ceased. The initial response package included NZ$600 million to support aviation (Twyford, 2020). There has been a focus on maintaining airfreight capacity and essential regional connections. With migration, there was a net gain of only 3,700 in the period April-October 2020, with 9000 New Zealand citizens returning as against 5200 non-New Zealanders departing (a reversal of the usual pattern whereby more New Zealanders departed); net migration in the 12 months to the end of October 2020 was 59,500, but 55,800 arrived before the imposition of restrictions in March 2020 (StatsNZ, 2020c).

Schools and institutions of higher education closed during the highest level of lockdown. Schools re-opened earlier than universities, but many of the latter had resumed on-campus activities by September-October. Although international students were less significant than in Australia (roughly 750,000 students in Australia compared to 100,000 in New Zealand), international education ranked as New Zealand's fourth most important export industry. New Zealand universities faced economic difficulties because of travel restrictions affecting international students, but so did the economy more broadly.

Re-positioning in international politics

While the pandemic has manifested itself most obviously at a domestic level in terms of public health and the economy, there are also many ways in which Australia and New Zealand have been affected internationally.

One element of international involvement has been in relation to global health politics. While there was some scapegoating of the World Health Organization in some quarters (most notably with President Trump), some of that body's alleged failures were due to slow action by members (China being slow to notify the WHO of details concerning the Wuhan outbreak). In April 2020 Australia was prominent in calls for an international inquiry into the origins and spread of COVID-19, leading to criticism from China. Subsequently the World Health Assembly at its meeting in May 2020 instituted such an inquiry, with Helen Clark (former New Zealand prime minister and former director of the United Nations Development Programme) appointed as co-chair.

Regionally the pandemic has led to increased Australian and New Zealand assistance to neighbouring developing countries. The pandemic has affected the Pacific island countries (PICs) but less so than in many regions of the world, with low case numbers but a major economic impact (see the articles on the Pacific island countries in this special issue). Indonesia, on the other hand, has been more strongly affected (and, with a population of about 270 million, has many more people); as of 16 December 2020, Indonesia had had 629,429 COVID cases, and 19,111 deaths (probably an underestimate) (figures from Worldometer).

Building on its existing programme for promoting regional health security (Australia has a designated ambassador in this area), Australia has established a series of 'partnerships for recovery' focused on the PICs and Timor-Leste to assist its regional neighbours in their response to the pandemic (Australian Government, Department of Foreign Affairs and Trade, 2020b). More broadly, Australia has supported the COVID-19 Vaccine Access and Health Security Program in Pacific and Southeast Asian countries. Support for infrastructure development has been expanded through the Australian Infrastructure Financing Facility for the Pacific, established previously as part of Australia's Pacific 'step up'. Although not counted officially as part of Australia's foreign aid, increased funding for the COVID-19 response package for the Pacific and Timor-Leste (A$305 million over two years in the federal budget of October 2020) has effectively increased the proportion of Australian GDP going to such aid, while also emphasising further the focus on these countries (under the Coalition government foreign aid had declined to about 2.0%) (Fox & Handley, 2020).

In the case of Indonesia, there was an initial 'step up' in Australian aid of A$21 million to deal with immediate issues arising from COVID (Australian Embassy, Indonesia, 2020); in the 2020–2021 federal budget total bilateral aid to Indonesia (not just for COVID-related matters) was set at A$255.7 million, and estimated total aid at A$299 million (including assistance through multilateral programmes); this figure was essentially the same as for 2019–2020 (Australian Government, Department of Foreign Affairs and Trade, 2020a). In real terms this meant a decline in Australian aid to Indonesia, even allowing for COVID (see further, Howes, 2020)

As with Australia, New Zealand's development assistance (almost 3.0% of GDP) concentrates on its Pacific neighbours. New Zealand has given additional support in this region in response to the pandemic, starting with a package of NZ$50 million (New Zealand, Ministry of Foreign Affairs and Trade, 2020). Matching Australia's Pacific 'step up', New Zealand has its Pacific Reset, with similar objectives. With 60% of New Zealand's aid going to the South Pacific, COVID has essentially meant some shift of focus, with greater emphasis on strengthening health systems and dealing with the economic impact; New Zealand has responded also to urgent requests relating to COVID in Indonesia and Timor-Leste (see further Kings, 2020). New Zealand has said it will act as an advocate to ensure the Pacific islands have access to a COVID vaccine when it becomes available (Powles, 2020, p. 12).

One element of the increased engagement by Australia and New Zealand in the South Pacific has been the need to ensure that their role remains more significant than that of China. China provided some assistance to the PICs in response to COVID, such as an initial US$1.9 million to fund medical supplies; it has also facilitated information-sharing and engaged in COVID diplomacy to draw attention to its positive role (Zhang, 2020). Overall, however, China's COVID role in the South Pacific is small compared with that of Australia and New Zealand.

Apart from the situation in the South Pacific, shifts in geopolitics in the Asia-Pacific arising from the pandemic affect Australia and New Zealand. China's relatively quick recovery from COVID has improved its position in terms of geopolitics (Bradsher, 2020); the US on the other hand has been weakened (for an argument to the contrary, see Drezner, 2020). Nevertheless, there have been some tensions in Sino-Australian relations, partly due to the pandemic, but more broadly relating to China's more assertive diplomacy in the region and Australia's high profile on some issues affecting China (perceived negatively by China, including the passage of foreign interference legislation). China has restricted the import of some items from Australia, such as barley, beef and lamb, cotton, timber, wine and lobsters, with coal also affected (Sullivan, 2020); Chinese students and tourists could not come to Australia because of COVID. Despite this bleak picture, given that normally about 30% of Australian trade is with China, Australia's overall trade with China at the beginning of August 2020 was reportedly 4.0% higher than at the comparable time in 2019, with increases in Australian exports of iron ore, grains and wool (Bagshaw, 2020). Insofar as Australia and New Zealand are relatively successful in combating COVID, one would expect some enhancement in the geopolitical importance of both powers, noting also the considerable 'soft power' of Prime Minister Jacinda Ardern (see further, Lowy Institute, 2020). In terms of relativities, however, we might note that China also was relatively successful in its response to the pandemic (despite COVID originating in China); according to Worldometer (16 December 2020), China ranked 207th for number of cases relative to population (better than Australia and New Zealand).

The future

The COVID pandemic has occasioned much thinking and debate about the future direction of both Australia and New Zealand. While at one level there has understandably been a prioritising of immediate health and economic issues arising from COVID, at another level there has been the view that the pandemic presents an opportunity for a 'reset' in relation to major policy issues confronting both countries. In terms of the financial commitment of both governments, the response to COVID has been compared to the mobilisation involved in fighting a major war. Just as there is a need post-war to determine priorities in reconstruction, so there is a need to think about what post-COVID reconstruction might entail.

In Australia, some edited books emanating from progressive (mainly Labor) circles emerged (Dawson & McCalman, 2020; Plibersek, 2020). Non-partisan think tanks such as the Lowy Institute (Edwards, 2020), the Australian Strategic Policy Institute (Coyne & Jennings, 2020; Shoebridge & Sharland, 2020) and the Grattan Institute were also very active. To take just one example, the book edited by Emma Dawson and Janet McCalman covered not just health and economic issues, but indigenous, environmental (climate change), educational and constitutional issues (including political process).

On the side of the federal government, its thinking emerged in the context of the policies it developed and implemented, the budget of October 2020 being a pre-eminent example. It also established a National COVID-19 Commission Advisory Board to provide a business perspective on economic recovery (announced 25 March 2020). While the federal government appeared strongly Keynesian in its economic response to the crisis, there was a question as to whether this would last in the long term.

In the initial phase of the pandemic there was some element of bipartisan cooperation in Australia, with the apparent suspension of 'politics as usual'. As time progressed there were more political tensions and more evident disagreements about the best balance between health and economic considerations in the anti-COVID strategy. (See further Murphy, 2020.)

Across the Tasman 'Saint' Jacinda, despite her international reputation, had had her pre-COVID domestic difficulties. She nevertheless surged ahead during the pandemic; the victory of the Labour Party in the national elections of 17 October confirming this perception. Labour under Ardern's leadership won an absolute majority of seats (64 seats, 49.1% of votes) (New Zealand, Electoral Commission, 2020), a very difficult feat in the mixed member proportional (MMP) system. With a majority Labour government, the constraints that exist with a coalition will not be present. New Zealand is in a more severe recession than is Australia. One can expect the second Ardern government to govern from the middle with practical, Keynesian-type measures.[3]

The success of Australia and New Zealand in their response to the pandemic (allowing for New Zealand's more severe recession) has positioned both countries to exert a stronger influence in the post-COVID world. While this will be most obvious in the South Pacific context, Australia at least should have a stronger voice in Asia-Pacific affairs; while Australia has its own bilateral tensions with China, Australia stands to benefit should there be some improvement in the atmospherics of Sino-US relations under the Biden administration (keeping in mind that this is not a foregone conclusion; there are likely to be some continuities with the policies of the Trump administration).

Conclusion

Summing up the experience of Australia and New Zealand in response to the pandemic, both countries have done relatively well in international terms, achieving high levels of suppression. New Zealand has done better than Australia in per capita terms, although the Australian figures are skewed by the impact of the second wave in Victoria. Without Victoria, the other Australian states and territories are roughly comparable to or even better than New Zealand (Queensland, South Australia, Western Australia, the Australian Capital Territory and the Northern Territory are better in per capita terms). In the Asia-Pacific, Japan and South Korea have been roughly comparable to Australia and New Zealand in their response to the pandemic; China and Taiwan have done better. Vietnam stands out among the developing countries for minimising COVID cases, although Thailand and Malaysia have also done well; Singapore was initially an exemplar but then fell behind.

The geographical isolation of Australia and New Zealand facilitated the strategies they adopted for combating COVID. Essentially all the jurisdictions in Australia and New Zealand aimed for assertive suppression, but with some variation in just how strong that was. New Zealand was aided by its unitary political system and Ardern's leadership. Strong political cooperation among the various jurisdictions in Australia subsequently became less so, with differences emerging between the federal government and the states, and among the Australian states. The second wave in Victoria exacerbated these tensions, but these eased with the ending of that wave. The centre-right of the political spectrum generally preferred some modifications in the strategy of assertive suppression.

Economically both Australia and New Zealand adopted Keynesian strategies in responding to the pandemic, injecting large sums to counter unemployment and to assist businesses. The level of debt is comparable to that undertaken by governments in wartime, the aim being to ensure that there is no economic collapse and to position the economy for subsequent revival.

Given that Australia and New Zealand have been relatively successful in international terms in combating COVID, there should be consequent gains in their geopolitical importance. This will be most obvious for both countries in relation to the South Pacific region; for Australia there should also be relative gains in relation to the broader Asia-Pacific.

Notes

1. The definition of essential services was broader in Australia than in New Zealand; New Zealand closed more non-essential services. Personal communication from Professor David Dunt, Melbourne School of Population and Global Health, University of Melbourne.
2. Personal communication from Professor David Dunt.
3. Note also the return of the Labor government in Queensland, with a clear victory in the state elections of 31 October 2020. Queensland has arguably been the most successful jurisdiction in the whole of Australia and New Zealand in combating COVID-19.

Acknowledgments

I wish to thank Professor David Dunt (Melbourne School of Population and Global Health, University of Melbourne), and Mr Connor O'Brien (School of Social and Political Sciences, University of Melbourne) for helpful feedback on an earlier version of this paper.

Disclosure statement

No potential conflict of interest was reported by the author.

ORCID

Derek McDougall http://orcid.org/0000-0003-1996-4240

References

Alcorn, G. (2020, September 9). 'Still stand with Dan?': Victorian premier's career will live or die by his coronavirus gamble, *Guardian Australia*, https://www.theguardian.com/australia-news/2020/sep/09/still-stand-with-dan-victorian-premiers-career-will-live-or-die-by-his-corona virus-gamble?

Australia, Royal Commission into Aged Care Quality and Safety. (2020). *Aged care and COVID-19: A special report.*https://agedcare.royalcommission.gov.au/sites/default/files/2020-10/aged-care-and-covid-19-a-special-report.pdf

Australian Bureau of Statistics. (2020a, September 2). *Economic activity fell 7.0 per cent in June quarter.* Media Release.https://www.abs.gov.au/media-centre/media-releases/economic-activity-fell-70-cent-june-quarter

Australian Bureau of Statistics. (2020b, July 16). *Labour force.*https://www.abs.gov.au/statistics/labour/employment-and-unemployment/labour-force-australia/jun-2020

Australian Bureau of Statistics. (2020c, September 24). *National, state and territory population.* https://www.abs.gov.au/statistics/people/population/national-state-and-territory-population/latest-release

Australian Bureau of Statistics. (2020d, December 2). *Economic activity increased 3.3% in September quarter.* Media Release.https://www.abs.gov.au/media-centre/media-releases/eco nomic-activity-increased-33-september-quarter

Australian Embassy, Indonesia. (2020, May 29). *Australia-Indonesia partnership to respond to COVID-19.*https://indonesia.embassy.gov.au/jakt/MR20_008.html

Australian Government. (2020). *Budget 2020-21.* Budget Overview. https://budget.gov.au/2020-21/content/overview.htm#top

Australian Government, Department of Foreign Affairs and Trade. (2020a). *Development partnership in Indonesia.* Overview of Australia's aid. https://www.dfat.gov.au/geo/indonesia/develop ment-assistance/Pages/development-assistance-in-indonesia

Australian Government, Department of Foreign Affairs and Trade. (2020b). *Partnerships for recovery: Australia's COVID-19 development response.* https://www.dfat.gov.au/sites/default/files/partnerships-for-recovery-australias-covid-19-development-response.pdf

Australian Government, Department of Health. (2020a, December 16). *Coronavirus (COVID-19) current situation and case numbers.* https://www.health.gov.au/news/health-alerts/novel-coronavirus-2019-ncov-health-alert/coronavirus-covid-19-current-situation-and-case-numbers

Australian Government, Department of Health. (2020b, December 11). *Australia's vaccine agreements.* https://www.health.gov.au/australias-vaccine-agreements

Bagshaw, E. (2020, August 4). Australian trade with China surges as rest of world falls. *Sydney Morning Herald.* https://www.smh.com.au/world/asia/australian-trade-with-china-surges-as-rest-of-the-world-falls-20200804-p55icy.html

Baker, M., Wilson, N., & Anglemyer, A. (2020, August 7). Successful elimination of COVID-19 transmission in New Zealand. *New England Journal of Medicine, 383*(8), e56. COVID-19 Notes Series. https://doi.org/10.1056/NEJMc2025203

Bradsher, K. (2020, October 18). With COVID-19 under control, China's economy surges ahead. *New York Times.* https://www.nytimes.com/2020/10/18/business/china-economy-covid.html

Colebatch, T. (2020, September 7). Most of the world would fail the Andrews test. *Inside Story.* https://insidestory.org.au/most-of-the-world-would-fail-the-andrews-test/

Coyne, & Jennings, P. (Eds.). (2020). *After COVID-19, vol. 1: Australia and the world re-build.* Australian Strategic Policy Institute.

Dawson, E., & McCalman, J. (Eds.). (2020). *What happens next? Reconstructing Australia after COVID-19.* Melbourne University Press.

A Doctors' Open Letter to Dan Andrews. (2020, September 1). *Quadrant online.* https://quadrant.org.au/opinion/qed/2020/09/a-doctors-open-letter-to-daniel-andrews/

Drezner, D. W. (2020). The song remains the same: International relations after COVID-19. *International Organization, 74*(Supplement), 1–18. https://doi.org/10.1017/S0020818320000351

Eaqub, S. (2020, May 15). Budget 2020: A massive spend-up but not transformational. Radio New Zealand, News, https://www.rnz.co.nz/news/on-the-inside/416701/budget-2020-a-massive-spend-up-but-not-transformational

Edwards, J. (2020, August 20). *The costs of COVID: Australia's economic prospects in a wounded world. analyses.* Lowy Institute. https://www.lowyinstitute.org/publications/costs-covid-australia-economic-prospects-wounded-world

Fox, L., & Handley. (2020, October 7). Australia's aid program increased to help Pacific neighbours fight COVID-19. ABC News. https://www.abc.net.au/news/2020-10-07/foreign-aid-budget-unofficial-increase-pacific-asia-covid-19/12737096

Gilbert, L., & Lilly, A. (2020, August 20). *Independent review, final report, Newmarch House COVID-19 outbreak (April-June 2020).* Australian Government, Department of Health. https://www.health.gov.au/sites/default/files/documents/2020/08/newmarch-house-covid-19-outbreak-independent-review-newmarch-house-covid-19-outbreak-independent-review-final-report.pdf

Hair, J. (2020, August 14). Ruby Princess inquiry slams 'inexcusable' mistakes made by NSW health, ABC News. https://www.abc.net.au/news/2020-08-14/ruby-princess-coronavirus-inquiry-findings-handed-down/12557714

Howes, S. (2020, October 7). *Total aid increased but cruel cuts outside the Pacific*, DevPolicyBlog, Development Policy Centre, Australian National University, https://devpolicy.org/2020-aid-budget-20201007/

Kings, J. (2020, May 8). *Pivoting New Zealand's aid programme to respond to COVID-19*, DevPolicyBlog, Development Policy Centre, Australian National University, https://devpolicy.org/pivoting-new-zealands-aid-programme-to-respond-to-covid-19-20200508-3/

Lowy Institute. (2020). *Lowy Institute Asia power index, 2020 edition.* https://power.lowyinstitute.org/

Michie, F. (2020, September 12). St Basil's chairman stands down as data shows 580 coronavirus aged care deaths, mainly in Victoria. ABC News. https://www.abc.net.au/news/2020-09-12/st-basils-chair-stands-down-federal-aged-care-coronavirus-deaths/12657134

The Morning Show. (2020, September 29). *Health Minister Greg Hunt 'confident' COVID available as early as January*, https://7news.com.au/the-morning-show/health-minister-greg-hunt-confident-covid-vaccine-available-as-early-as-january-c-1348558
Murphy, K. (2020). The end of certainty: Scott Morrison and pandemic politics. *Quarterly Essay*, 79. https://www.quarterlyessay.com.au/essay/2020/09/the-end-of-certainty
New Zealand, Electoral Commission. (2020). *2020 general election and referendums -preliminary count.* https://www.electionresults.govt.nz/electionresults_2020_preliminary/
New Zealand, Ministry of Foreign Affairs and Trade. (2020). *Peace, rights & security, COVID-19 response and recovery.*https://www.mfat.govt.nz/en/peace-rights-and-security/covid-19-response-and-recovery/#pacific
New Zealand, Ministry of Health. (2020, December 16). *COVID-19: Current cases.*https://www.health.govt.nz/our-work/diseases-and-conditions/covid-19-novel-coronavirus/covid-19-data-and-statistics/covid-19-current-cases#summary
Plibersek, T. (Ed.). (2020). *Upturn: A better normal after COVID-19.* NewSouth Books.
Powles, A. (2020). New Zealand's COVID-19 support to the Pacific islands. In M. Shoebridge & L. Sharland (Eds.), *After COVID-19, vol. 2: Australia, the region and multilateralism* (pp. 11–15). Australian Strategic Policy Institute.
Remeikis, A. (2020, October 19). COVID rewrites Australia's future, with huge drop in population signalling challenges ahead. *The Guardian.* https://www.theguardian.com/business/2020/oct/19/covid-rewrites-australias-future-with-huge-drop-in-population-signalling-challenges-ahead
Robertson, G. (2020, March 17). *$12.1 billion support for New Zealanders and business.* Ministerial Releases. https://www.beehive.govt.nz/release/121-billion-support-new-zealanders-and-business
Rollason, B., & Staff. (2020, October 15). Victoria's COVID-19 response leaves state budget billions of dollars in deficit. ABC News. https://www.abc.net.au/news/2020-10-15/victoria-records-first-budget-deficit-in-nearly-three-decades/12769524
Roy, E. A. (2020, September 17). New Zealand in COVID recession after worst quarterly GDP fall on record. *The Guardian.* https://www.theguardian.com/world/2020/sep/17/new-zealand-in-covid-recession-after-worst-quarterly-gdp-fall-on-record
Shoebridge, M., & Sharland, L. (Eds.). (2020). *After COVID-19, vol. 2: Australia, the region and multilateralism.* Australian Strategic Policy Institute.
StatsNZ. (2020a, August 5). *COVID-19 lockdown has widespread effects on labour market.*https://www.stats.govt.nz/news/covid-19-lockdown-has-widespread-effects-on-labour-market
StatsNZ. (2020b, November 17). *Estimated population of NZ.* https://www.stats.govt.nz/indicators/population-of-nz
StatsNZ. (2020c, December 14) *More departures than arrivals since March.* https://www.stats.govt.nz/news/more-departures-than-arrivals-since-march
Strongman, S. (2020). *COVID-19 timeline: How the pandemic started, spread and stalled life in New Zealand.* Radio New Zealand. https://shorthand.radionz.co.nz/coronavirus-timeline/
Sullivan, K. (2020, December 17). China's list of sanctions and tariffs on Australian trade is growing. Here's what has been hit so far. ABC News. https://www.abc.net.au/news/2020-12-17/australian-trade-tension-sanctions-china-growing-commodities/12984218
Ting, I., & Palmer, A. (2020, May 4, updated 5 May). One hundred days of the coronavirus. ABC News. https://www.abc.net.au/news/2020-05-04/charting-100-days-of-the-coronavirus-crisis-in-australia/12197884?nw=0
Truu, M. (2020, May 1). Australia's migration intake to fall 85 per cent due to coronavirus, Scott Morrison says. SBS News. https://www.sbs.com.au/news/australia-s-migration-intake-to-fall-85-per-cent-due-to-coronavirus-scott-morrison-says
Twyford, P. (2020, March 19) *Govt announces aviation relief package.* Ministerial Releases. https://www.beehive.govt.nz/release/govt-announces-aviation-relief-package
Victoria, COVID-19 Hotel Quarantine Inquiry. (2020, December 21). Final report and recommendations, Vol. I & II. *Parliamentary papers nos. 191 and 192 (2018–2020).* Victorian government.

Victoria, Department of Health and Human Services. (2020, December 15). *Coronavirus (COVID-19) daily update*.https://www.dhhs.vic.gov.au/coronavirus-covid-19-daily-update

Worldometer. (2020). COVID-19 Coronavirus pandemic, reported cases and deaths by country or territory.https://www.worldometers.info/coronavirus/#countries

Zhang, D. (2020). China's coronavirus 'COVID-19 diplomacy' in the Pacific. *In Brief, 2020/10*. Department of Pacific Affairs. Australian National University. http://dpa.bellschool.anu.edu.au/sites/default/files/publications/attachments/2020-04/ib_2020_10_zhang_final_0.pdf

COVID-19 in the Pacific Island Commonwealth: microstates managing a macro-challenge

Richard Herr

ABSTRACT
Although the heritage and values of the Commonwealth of Nations are integrally woven into the political DNA of the Pacific Island region, this connection is not directly evident in the robust ecology of multilateral organisations that have developed over the past 80 years or in meeting the challenge of COVID-19. The region's small states have responded nationally rather than regionally. With only a limited exposure to the disease itself, these small states have been comprehensively impacted economically by COVID-19. Border closures as well as the suspension of significant transport options reduced income from tourists and other travellers. Economic conditions reduced the demand for the region's exports while diminished imports cut national income from customs and excises. The use of stimulus packages and borrowings to keep people employed is both necessary and a risk. It could prove ill-advised if tourists and markets do not return to pre-COVID levels. This article looks at the impact of the pandemic in, and on, the region and at some of the factors that might shape the post-COVID order for the Commonwealth's Pacific Island members.

Introduction

COVID-19 (hereinafter referred to as 'COVID') has tied the Pacific Island Commonwealth states to the rest of the world like few other events. Despite only a limited exposure to the disease itself, these small states have been comprehensively impacted by the global pandemic. Through the first seven months of the pandemic in 2020, however, it has been the economic damage more than the disease itself which has harmed Pacific populations. This assessment may be subject to change as the effects of the stress on mental health and the effects of missed or delayed treatments become evident in the future. Nonetheless, COVID's economic impact has been evident from the outset. Border closures as well as the suspension of significant transport options reduced income from tourists and other travellers. Economic conditions reduced the demand for the region's exports while diminished imports cut national income from customs and excises. Reduced trade even threatened food security as many islands depend on imports for basic food stuffs.

While the challenges of coping with COVID are far from over, concerns over both the transition to and nature of the post-pandemic Pacific are already a matter of speculation and creative thinking. Key decisions on how to manage current scarce resources to meet present demands wisely depend on the expectations of what will speed an effective transition to the world after COVID. The transformation of COVID from a pandemic into an endemic condition is far from clear in terms of timing and severity. The Commonwealth Pacific states appear to have adopted the 'old normal' as a default position for the post-COVID 'new normal'. Given that these small states cannot have a significant role in shaping the post-COVID order, this may be the only posture they can adopt. Yet, the use of stimulus packages and borrowings to keep their people employed to return to pre-COVID jobs and industries could prove to have been ill-advised if tourists, other travellers and markets do not return to pre-COVID levels. Airline capacity cuts, new consumption patterns and deskilled populations may not be easily reversible even in the middle term. This article looks at the impact of the pandemic in, and on, the region and at some of the factors that might shape the post-COVID order for the Commonwealth's Pacific Island members.

The Commonwealth in the Pacific Islands

Excluding Australia and New Zealand, insularity, small size, developing economic status and remoteness are key descriptors for the other nine Commonwealth members in the southern Pacific Ocean.[1] Only the largest of these nine, Papua New Guinea (PNG), has a land border which it shares with Indonesia. PNG is also the only member with a population greater than one million. All are developing states that became eligible for membership through the experience of colonialism but not all were British colonies. A minority were scions of Australia or New Zealand. Due to a troubled history of coups, Fiji has been suspended and re-joined several times and was most recently reinstated in 2014. These states are located in a region whose midpoint is the most remote of any inhabited region from major global concentrations of population. These essential characteristics of the Pacific Islands region have very much framed the impact of the COVID-19 pandemic in the Commonwealth Pacific.

The value of the Commonwealth to the conduct of regional relations, including the response to the COVID pandemic, is rather difficult to calculate. Potentially, the Commonwealth network could play a central part in organising the regional agenda. Yet, although the members of the Commonwealth constitute a majority of the membership in the main Pacific Island regional organisations, the Commonwealth members do not caucus as an association within these bodies. In the half century since Pacific Island states began joining the Commonwealth, this system has developed in parallel to the robust interrelated regional system of intergovernmental organisations that formulate, coordinate and implement a wide range of policy across more than a score of island states and territories (Herr & Bergin, 2011).

There are two principal reasons that may explain the absence of subregional caucusing by the Pacific Island Commonwealth states – as members of the Commonwealth. The primary reason is the leadership role historically played by Commonwealth countries in constructing the region's architecture. Australia and New Zealand in 1944 initiated the process leading to the Pacific Community (SPC) which today is the region's premier technical development body.[2] The independent countries that established the Pacific Islands Forum (PIF) in 1971 as their summit level mechanism for political cooperation and coordination were members of the Commonwealth or in line to become Commonwealth eligible.[3] Thus Commonwealth ties and values, in a real sense, were hardwired into the DNA of the regional system. Yet with some irony, the second reason for the lack of a robust and visible role for the Commonwealth brand has been the perceived need to avoid alienating non-Commonwealth countries. This was particularly compelling within the SPC. From its origins, it has been important to Australia and New Zealand that France and the US be engaged in the regional system both for their own international standing as well as for their territories in the region.

COVID-19 at the region's gate

Regional preparations to deal with COVID were begun in January 2020 (World Health Organization [WHO], 2020a). This was well before the World Health Organization (WHO) officially characterised COVID as a pandemic on March 11 (2020b). Just over a week later, two Commonwealth countries reported their first case of COVID. Fiji reported its case on March 19 and PNG reported its first case the following day on March 20. Subsequently, to late September 2020, only four other Pacific Island countries – Commonwealth of the Northern Marianas (CNMI), French Polynesia, Guam and New Caledonia have reported cases. The COVID figures have been in flux for the Pacific Island states and territories over the course of this research. However, a snapshot of these numbers in September 2020 gives a fair picture of the course of the disease in the first six months of the pandemic. As of 22 September 2020, the 6 countries together have reported 4,194 cases and 48 deaths. PNG accounted for 534 cases and 7 deaths and Fiji 32 cases with two deaths. Guam has dominated overwhelmingly in the number of cases and deaths with 3,225 and 40 respectively. Thus, in global terms, the Pacific Island region has protected itself very effectively from the first wave of the pandemic.[4]

There have been some important factors that contributed to this success. The region's geography has been a very significant influence. Insularity has conferred a natural advantage by making external transmission more easily controlled for all states except for PNG which does have a somewhat porous land border. The benefit of insularity has been reinforced by geographic remoteness. Unlike a compact region of islands like the Caribbean area, in the Pacific Island region travelling to, and within, the region involves very significant distances. These factors explain why the bulk of the cases in the South Pacific have been limited to countries with substantial international traffic such as tourism. The majority of the region's polities do not engage directly with global pandemic hotspots. The CNMI, Fiji, French Polynesia, Guam, and New Caledonia have important tourism industries, but Guam's figures have been particularly impacted by its large US military facilities.

Arguably, the Islands' policy decisions on restricting travel and closing borders were made less domestically controversial as international travel into the region was cut off at source. Not only did Australia, New Zealand and other states restrict their international flights, but quarantining travellers at transit or entry points into the region discouraged using what access was available. Such actions certainly contributed to the effectiveness of government action by Palau and Vanuatu which made them something of COVID outliers despite their dependence on tourism. While not yet needed, geography could have played a part in limiting the spread of COVID internally. All regional states and territories are archipelagic except for Guam and Niue. This would help in isolating hotspots domestically if the international borders were breached.

National responses to the pandemic

COVID-19 has been first and foremost a threat to the health of Pacific Islanders but the national effectiveness in blunting the intrusion of the disease has meant the principal impact over the course of 2020 has been to their economies. Nevertheless, the trajectory of the crisis was far from evident in January. The SPC warned early that it did not believe its members could cope well if large numbers were infected by the disease due to the 'lack of infrastructure, equipment, and qualified personnel.' (SPC, 2020). Equally worryingly, the SPC noted that most members did not have the necessary laboratory equipment to process tests for identifying cases making it necessary to send samples to other countries for analysis. For the Commonwealth states this meant sending to Australia or New Zealand.

Thus, the first priority for all states and territories was to secure the time to obtain the capacity to meet the expected demands on their public health systems. Given their limited resources and medical capacities, the initial step was prophylaxis followed by a search for increased medical equipment, supplies and reserves.

As the International Monetary Fund (2020a) documents in its Global Review of COVID Policy Responses, the initial public health response to COVID was fairly similar across the Commonwealth Pacific. All imposed border restrictions – air and sea – by mid-March 2020. Samoa was the first to impose its travel restrictions in January motivated to act early by the deadly measles epidemic only months before. The closure of international airports, quarantining of cruising yachts, restrictions on domestic travel along with limiting public gatherings, closures of schools and businesses also were typical responses although these measures varied in duration and completeness. It was necessary to keep transport avenues open to some degree to accommodate other health related measures such as delivering medical supplies, facilitating testing, and maintaining food stocks.

Fiji pursued the most aggressive measures amongst the Commonwealth Pacific states because it was the first to directly experience the disease. The Government imposed a nationwide curfew and lockdowns of affected areas in March and April. The first lockdown centred on Lautoka and included door-to-door screening (body temperature checks) of the entire population within the city by the Fiji military. By July, Fiji had no active cases and felt secure enough with its testing and quarantine measures to allow the repatriation of citizens trapped abroad. PNG followed a similar trajectory with a national shut down in March and a state of emergency declaration imposing significant internal restrictions. However, when this ended in June, there was a serious resurgence of COVID cases which seems to have originated in a hospital and testing facility in Port Moresby. This spike appears to have abated by early September.

There is a familiar albeit tragic irony for the Pacific microstates that the measures taken outside the region have magnified consequences within the region. The steps taken internationally to contain the spread of COVID have served to reinforce actions taken by the Pacific Island states to protect their physical health. However, the economic effects have been disproportionally devastating for a region of developing states with a high level of vulnerability. The collapse of international tourism, the barriers to labour mobility, the job losses in diaspora host countries, and contraction of development projects have all served to amplify the economic consequences of national measures to pursue prophylactic strategies against the disease. Thus, virtually concomitantly with the health measures, the Pacific Island states have had to follow the lead of their developed neighbours and pursue offsetting economic strategies but without their financial reserves or inherent robustness.

All of the Pacific Commonwealth states have suffered a severe downturn in revenues with the falloff in customs, excises and tax income. Nauru has been an apparent exception since fish licences and aid financed developments seem to have blunted the worst of COVID's economic impact for this minuscule nation. The other countries, faring less well, have legislated economic stimulus programmes although these might be better styled relief measures. They basically are intended to reduce the consequences of unemployment, business closures and reduced family support from overseas relations in addition to meeting national urgent balance of payment needs. Financing these measures has involved borrowing against national superannuation funds and from international institutions such as ADB and IMF as well as eating into national currency reserves. New debts and reduced national capacity will make the post-COVID economic recovery far more challenging for these small states than their wealthier neighbours better able to afford their domestic stimulus packages.

The stimulus packages have only moderated, not obviated, the need for national belt-tightening. COVID-related budget cuts have forced a reduction in some government services despite the greater demand for services. Some cuts appear counterproductive because they are likely to frustrate the return to a pre-COVID normal. A Hobson's choice was forced on Fiji with regard to its majority-owned Fiji Airways. Notwithstanding the centrality of tourism to the national income and airline's importance to generating Fiji's tourist visits, nearly 800 jobs were terminated including the contracts of all expatriate pilots in May (Narayan, 2020). At a time when Asia-Pacific relations will be significant in rebuilding the post-COVID economic order, the Fijian Government announced it would close its missions in Brussels, Kuala Lumpur, Port Moresby, Seoul and Washington permanently as an economic measure. The Minister of Economy, Aiyaz Sayed-Khaiyum defended the budget decision that these missions 'do not reliably make returns on Government's investment in their operations' (Vula, 2020).

The economic responses of Pacific Commonwealth countries to COVID have been coloured by exogenous events. In the case of Samoa, the economic effects of the measles epidemic had scarcely begun to be addressed before the pandemic deepened the government's financial hole making necessary an urgent IMF loan (IMF, Press Release 20/189). For Vanuatu, it was dealing with cleaning up after Tropical Cyclone Harold hit in early April as well as the loss of significant income from seasonal workers excluded from Australia by border closures. PNG's uniqueness amongst the Pacific Commonwealth countries in having a land border has meant that enforcement of frontier controls is not entirely in its own hands. This has forced more costly, and initially less effective, measures to guard the Western Province border as well as closer cooperation with Indonesia (Blades, 2020).

Insofar as the economic stimulus packages have served to provide relief for unemployment and business losses, they may have ameliorated some of the social pain inflicted on Pacific societies. Self-help has shown some success in bridging the gap. Home garden schemes, sometimes with government support, have become common. Social media has promoted the cashless economy through facilitating barter arrangements in Fiji, PNG, Samoa, Solomon Islands, Tonga and Vanuatu with some notable success (Tora, 2020). Indeed, Fiji's system, Barter for Better Fiji, was among a number of NGO activities selected by the UNDP for easing the social and economic impact of COVID (Chand, 2020). Despite such attempts to soften the economic pain of the pandemic, the effects on mental health, domestic violence and related concerns have grown as lockdowns and isolation have put families and individuals into a social pressure cooker (WHO, 2020c). An extensive gamut of social issues will be added to the inventory of unmet economic need as part of all regional post-COVID agendas.

International cooperation

Regionalism has long been important to the small states of the Pacific in helping to overcome their geographic challenges. Having effective regional relations and institutions also serves as a solid networking platform for extra-regional actors including multilateral agencies to reach even the remotest and smallest of the Pacific states. The value of the Pacific Island regional system in both directions has been well demonstrated in responding to the COVID pandemic.

The Pacific Community (SPC) has been the leading agency in setting the regional agenda on health and coordinating responses for its member states and territories having had health and medicine as a core mandate since its establishment in 1947. The SPC partnered with WHO in 1996 to establish the Pacific Public Health Surveillance Network (PPHSN) which has a specific mandate to monitor communicable diseases, 'especially those prone to outbreak' (WHO, 2020d). The SPC has served as the permanent focal point for the PPHSN. The SPC is proving its value to the Pacific Island region by facilitating a rapid response to the COVID pandemic both in its own right and serving as the principal regional partner for WHO.

In late January 2020, a Joint Incident Management Team (JIMT) was established by WHO and its PPHSN partners with WHO designated as the coordinating agency. In collaboration with the regional states, major donors and regional agencies, the JIMT developed a six-month 'Pacific Action Plan for 2019 Novel Coronavirus (COVID-19) Preparedness and Response'. Funding and logistics for implementing this plan was provided primarily by the two leading regional Commonwealth states, Australia and New Zealand. Critically in the first months of the pandemic, the Pacific Action Plan included providing national testing capacity to virtually all the Island states and territories. However, given national border closures, delivering this assistance required joint national agreements across the region to allow aid into the countries needing testing capacity. The Pacific Islands Forum leaders invoked their 2000 Biketawa Declaration, a broad security agreement, to establish a 'Pacific Humanitarian Pathway on COVID-19' in April 2020 to circumvent some of the obstacles created by the border closures. The Pathway has enabled a range of countries and agencies to coordinate and facilitate COVID-related assistance swiftly and safely (Pacific Islands Forum Secretariat [PIFS], 2020a).

Fortunately, the preventative measures taken so quickly before COVID took hold in the region obviated the need for some of the volume of medical supplies and health equipment that the Pacific Humanitarian Pathway was expected to facilitate. Nevertheless, there was a sense of competition in some quarters to meet the presumed demand. Much was made of China's putative 'mask diplomacy' in the early months of the pandemic. The global shortage of hospital supplies, testing equipment and respiratory aids was encapsulated in the need for protective face masks. Geopolitical concerns were raised by security analysts that China would use its manufacturing strength in this area to win a strategic 'hearts and minds' advantage burnishing its image as a responsible global leader (Wong, 2020). Questioning China's motives with regard to mask diplomacy in the Pacific Islands has been deepened by the perception in recent years that the PRC has been using just such soft power tactics for direct strategic advantage (Herr, 2019).

The road to recovery: from pandemic to endemic

Some seven months into the COVID pandemic, the Commonwealth's small Pacific states have suffered the economic consequences with their related social damage more than the destructive health effects of the disease. Essentially these states have escaped the virus at the expense of their economies. Nevertheless, COVID-19 continues to swirl all around them with all its menacing lethality should the disease breach their border defences. The way out of this predicament is not in the hands of the regional states. All but PNG can be described as living within a national 'bubble' protecting their people's health within as long as the bubble is not allowed to burst. The prevalence of the disease in so much of the rest of the world makes the Pacific Islands hostage to the global management of the pandemic. Yet, their bubbles' fragile protective membrane prevents the Pacific countries' return to economic health so long as the national bubble strategy frustrates international mobility.

The strategy for the hardest COVID-affected parts of the world appears to be to develop the mix of therapeutics and vaccines that turn the disease from a pandemic into a manageable endemic condition rather like the seasonal flu. It would still be deadly but medical and social protocols would be developed that could allow states to carry on in a way that feels 'normal' perhaps even the pre-COVID normal. However, the metrics that would enable rational and acceptable policies to navigate the period of this transition is very much a subject of partisan debate in the states most critically affected by the disease. How reliable the therapeutics, how effective the yet-to-be developed vaccines, how many deaths would be acceptable and how long a transition is needed? The answers to these questions will largely determine when, at a global level, it will be safe to reopen borders without quarantines, isolations, testing, closures and lockdowns. And, as ever, the Pacific Island states, will be the recipients of the decisions made elsewhere; unable to have an effective say in their determination.

Consideration of some transition to an endemic COVID condition has added another twist to the earlier geopolitical concerns over mask diplomacy. The small size of the Pacific Commonwealth states makes it technically feasible for these states to swing directly from being besieged by COVID as a pandemic to a relatively protected endemic stage. 'Vaccine diplomacy' is now on the table for leveraging influence given the advances China has made with its research and development (Massola, 2020). Immunising the microstates of the Pacific could well be within the resources of China if it develops a safe and effective vaccine before other vaccines become available. Whether vaccine diplomacy is even an option will depend on supply, demand and if there is a chokehold on distribution. Australia has countered by supporting several schemes to guarantee access to vaccines in sufficient amount to ensure availability in the Pacific Islands (Indo-Pacific Centre for Health Security, 2020). New Zealand is also engaged with these arrangements.

There are some interim measures being considered that could allow the Pacific states to turn their COVID-safe national bubbles into an asset regionally. The Commonwealth Pacific Island countries believe that their COVID status entitles them to be included in a travel bubble with either or, preferably, both Australia and New Zealand. As early as June 2020, Fiji proposed a partial and one-sided travel bubble with Australia to allow visitors and yachts *inter alia* to spend some time at limited destinations with careful health protocols (McIlroy, 2020). Their two developed Commonwealth partners have agreed to create a trans-Tasman bubble when feasible (Ross, 2020). The benefit of these proposals is to free visitors and workers from the need to undertake expensive quarantine requirements, but they will have to be effective both ways to really open up business and tourist traffic. The demand for seasonal labour during the austral summer and autumn in both Australia and New Zealand has been building pressure domestically in the two countries for the travel bubble while the need for the guest workers income is amplifying the lobbying from the Islands.

The Pacific Island states' success with containing the health threat has made the damage to their economies stand out more starkly as they look to recovery. Thus, if COVID is to have any geopolitical rebalancing consequences in the South Pacific, it is less likely to be a result of overwhelming Chinese medical largesse than the pandemic's geo-economic fallout. Estimates of a decline of 5.9% in regional real GDP and an increase in extreme poverty by 40% are compounded by the debt incurred to stave off the worst of the business and social impacts of these losses (Shen, 2020). The regional response has been led by the PIF Economic Ministers who endorsed a proposal at their 2020 meeting to establish a 'regional COVID-19 Economic Recovery Taskforce to lead a coordinated response for national and regional economic priorities both in meeting the pandemic setbacks and in the post-COVID recovery phase' (PIFS, 2020b).

The Taskforce faces some extremely serious challenges. Despite the G20's agreement for a 'debt standstill' to the end of 2020 for developing states and other measures to manage the Pacific Island states debt repayments, the threat of defaulting on international borrowings hangs like a sword of Damocles over most of the COVID-ravished economies of these states (Dyart & Rajah, 2020). The evidence that China can pursue strategic ambitions through leveraging COVID to secure a geo-economic transformation of the region, however, is mixed even if the ambition has substance (Kemish, 2020). Some point to the effects of COVID on China's economy as a likely limiting factor (Zhang, 2020). Moreover, the last two years suggest that the PRC has lost some enthusiasm for buying influence in the region (Pryke & Alexandre, 2020). The small Pacific Commonwealth states like the rest of the region will find their inherent vulnerability fully tested on the path to economic recovery. The engine of global revival will not pull with even and equal effect around the world. The restoration of economic growth is likely to be rather 'clunky' as different cars in the global train start up at different times with different levels of power to pull the following cars.

Unfortunately, the small Pacific states can be characterised as the caboose on a global economic freight train. The Islands' economic revival will depend very much on how quickly and with how much energy their traditional partners and markets restart their economies. Before the tourists return, for example, travellers in the source countries will need the disposable income and confidence to book vacations. Airlines and cruise ships will want to see reinvigorated demand to fully restore their services as will the travel agents, hotels and the myriad other elements of the travel industry. Similar factors will apply to international demand for the region's exports and the availability of its imports. Their small size may make some temporary economic boosts possible to soften the length of time it will take for global recovery to fully include the Pacific Islands. Nevertheless, sustainable economic activity in the region will depend on sustained international revitalisation.

Conclusions

The Commonwealth has not been overtly an organising influence in meeting the threat of COVID as the pandemic has beset the region, despite the political heritage and complexion of the small island states of the South Pacific that make this a profoundly Commonwealth region. Yet the sinews of the regional system and the strength of bilateral relations derive from deeply held Commonwealth sentiments. Australia and Zealand have taken a leadership role bilaterally, regionally and globally in seeking solutions for the sufferings COVID has inflicted on their fellow Commonwealth states. These small states have accepted a great deal of responsibility themselves for meeting the COVID challenge. They have closed their borders and imposed strict internal measures when necessary notwithstanding the economic consequences. They have also developed and empowered regional solutions through the regional organisations such as the SPC and PIF that serve to give them ownership of the regional response to the pandemic. Their shared Commonwealth values may well be decisive in determining the nature and extent of any remodelling of Pacific relations as a consequence of the damage traceable to COVID. Australia and New Zealand will be leaning on these Commonwealth values to limit any perceived adverse geopolitical changes.

Notes

1. The nine Pacific Island states members in order of their entry into the Commonwealth are: Nauru (1968); Fiji, Samoa and Tonga (all in 1970); PNG (1975), the Solomon Islands and Tuvalu (both in (1978); Kiribati (1979) and Vanuatu (1980). Two countries – the Cook Islands and Niue – enjoy an involvement with many Commonwealth activities but are ineligible being in a freely associated relationship with New Zealand.
2. Today the SPC's membership consists of 22 Pacific nations and territories (American Samoa, Cook Islands, Federated States of Micronesia, Fiji, French Polynesia, Guam, Kiribati, Marshall Islands, Nauru, New Caledonia, Niue, Northern Mariana Islands, Palau, Papua New Guinea, Pitcairn Islands, Samoa, Solomon Islands, Tokelau, Tonga, Tuvalu, Vanuatu, and Wallis and Futuna) and five of the six founding members (Australia, France, New Zealand, the UK and the US).
3. The PIF members are Australia, Cook Islands, Fiji, Federated States of Micronesia, Kiribati, Marshall Islands, Nauru, New Zealand, Niue, Palau, Papua New Guinea, Samoa, Solomon Islands, Tonga, Tuvalu and Vanuatu. French Polynesia and New Caledonia were admitted as full members in 2016.
4. Since this article went to review, the incidence of COVID in the region has changed slightly. New cases have been reported in American Samoa, Republic of the Marshall Islands, Solomon Islands, Vanuatu and Wallis and Futuna. These have not altered the fundaments of the limited health impact in the region. The cases appear to arise mainly from opening borders for repatriation. Those infected were quarantined under the protocols for repatriation without giving rising to community spread to date.

Disclosure statement

No potential conflict of interest was reported by the author.

References

Blades, J. (2020, April 24). Pandemic exposes weakness of PNG's border security. *Radio New Zealand*. https://www.rnz.co.nz/international/pacific-news/415003/pandemic-exposes-weakness-of-png-s-border-security

Chand, A. (2020, June 2). Six Fijian initiatives win grants from UNDP. *Fiji Times*. https://www.fijitimes.com/six-fijian-initiatives-win-grants-from-undp/

Dyart, A., & Rajah, R. (2020, June 4). Aiding the Pacific during Covid – A stock-take and further steps. *The Interpreter*. Lowy Institute. https://www.lowyinstitute.org/the-interpreter/aiding-pacific-during-covid-stock-take-and-further-steps

Herr, R. (2019, April). *Chinese influence in the Pacific Islands: The yin and yang of Soft Power*. Australian Strategic Policy Institute. https://www.aspi.org.au/report/chinese-influence-pacific-islands

Herr, R., & Bergin, A. (2011, November). *Our near abroad: Australia and Pacific islands regionalism*. Australian Strategic Policy Institute, Strategy Report. https://www.aspi.org.au/report/our-near-abroad-australia-and-pacific-islands-regionalism

Indo-Pacific Centre for Health Security. (2020, August 26). *Australia to promote COVID-19 vaccine equity for developing countries*. https://indopacifichealthsecurity.dfat.gov.au/australia-promote-covid-19-vaccine-equity-developing-countries

International Monetary Fund. (2020a). *Policy responses to COVID-19*. https://www.imf.org/en/Topics/imf-and-covid19/Policy-Responses-to-COVID-19

International Monetary Fund. (2020b). *Press release no. 20/189*. https://www.imf.org/en/News/Articles/2020/04/24/pr20189-samoa-imf-executive-board-approves-us-million-disbursement-address-covid-19-pandemic

Kemish, I. (2020, August 31). China wants to be a friend to the Pacific, but so far, it has failed to match Australia's COVID-19 response'. *The Conversation*. https://theconversation.com/china-wants-to-be-a-friend-to-the-pacific-but-so-far-it-has-failed-to-match-australias-covid-19-response-144911

Massola, J. (2020, October 11). Vaccine diplomacy offers risks and rewards for rising superpower. *Sydney Morning Herald*. https://www.smh.com.au/world/asia/vaccine-diplomacy-offers-risks-and-rewards-for-rising-superpower-20201007-p562zr.html

McIlroy, T. (2020, June 21). Fiji to open borders to Aussies and Kiwis in 'Bula Bubble' plan. *Australian Financial Review*. https://www.afr.com/politics/federal/fiji-to-open-borders-to-aussies-and-kiwis-in-bula-bubble-plan-20200621-p554p1

Narayan, V. (2020, May 25). Fiji Airways terminates contracts of 758 employees. *fijivillage*. https://www.fijivillage.com/news/Fiji-Airways-terminates-contracts-of-758-employees-lets-go-of-all-expat-pilots-and-some-expat-managers-and-implements-20-pay-cut-National-carrier-to-raise-debt-finance-to-ensure-survival-r5fx48/

Pacific Islands Forum Secretariat. (2020a, April 8). *Pacific Islands Forum Foreign Ministers agree to establish a Pacific Humanitarian pathway on COVID –19*. https://www.forumsec.org/2020/04/08/pacific-islands-forum-foreign-ministers-agree-to-establish-a-pacific-humanitarian-pathway-on-covid-19/

Pacific Islands Forum Secretariat. (2020b, August 13). *Forum Economic Ministers meeting outcomes document and statement on COVID-19*. https://www.forumsec.org/2020/08/14/2020-forum-economic-ministers-meeting-outcomes-document-and-statement-on-covid-19/

Pryke, J., & Alexandre, D. (2020, October 15). The Pacific has pulled off a coronavirus miracle. But it comes at a price. *Australian Broadcasting Corporation News*. https://www.abc.net.au/news/2020-10-15/coronavirus-pacific-economy-foriegn-aid-china/12754068

Ross, D. (2020, September 30). Jacinda Ardern suggests trans-Tasman bubble is near. *The Australian*. https://www.theaustralian.com.au/world/jacinda-ardern-suggests-transtasman-bubble-is-near/news-story/3e0d0b7979728fa77763f58f600853e7

Shen, K. (2020, September 9). *The economic costs of the pandemic for the Pacific Islands*. Center for Strategic and International Studies https://www.csis.org/blogs/new-perspectives-asia/economic-costs-pandemic-pacific-islands

SPC. (2020, March 20). *Update: COVID-19. https://php.spc.int/news/2020/03/spc-update-covid–19*

Tora, T. (2020, May 7). Two piglets for a Kayak: Fiji returns to Barter system as Covid-19 hits economy. *The Guardian*. https://www.theguardian.com/world/2020/may/08/two-piglets-for-a-kayak-fiji-returns-to-barter-system-as-covid-19-hits-economy

Vula, T. (2020, July 17). Budget 2020-2021: $8m cut across foreign missions; five embassies close permanently. *Fiji Times*. https://www.fijitimes.com/budget-2020-2021-8m-cut-across-foreign-missions-five-embassies-close-permanently/

Wong, B. (2020, March 25). China's mask diplomacy. *The Diplomat*. https://thediplomat.com/2020/03/chinas-mask-diplomacy/

World Health Organization. (2020a, June 11). *Engaging communities to prepare for COVID-19*. https://www.who.int/fiji/news/feature-stories/detail/defending-the-pacific

World Health Organization. (2020b, July 31). Rolling updates on coronavirus disease (COVID-19). *Events as they happen*. https://www.who.int/emergencies/diseases/novel-coronavirus-2019/events-as-they-happen

World Health Organization. (2020c, October 10). *Mental health in the Pacific, World Health Organization, 2020*. https://www.who.int/tokelau/news/detail/10-10-2020-mental-health-in-the-pacific

World Health Organization. (2020d). *The Pacific Public Health Surveillance Network (PPHSN)*. https://www.who.int/westernpacific/about/how-we-work/pacific-support/pphsn

Zhang, D. (2020, 10). China's Coronavirus 'COVID-19 diplomacy' in the Pacific. *In Brief*. Dept. of Pacific Affairs, Research School of Pacific and Asian Studies, The Australian National University. http://dpa.bellschool.anu.edu.au/sites/default/files/publications/attachments/2020-04/ib_2020_10_zhang_final_0.pdf

COVID-19 and tourism in Pacific SIDS: lessons from Fiji, Vanuatu and Samoa?

John Connell

ABSTRACT

Tourism was of critical economic importance in Pacific SIDS until COVID-19 border closures cut off international ties. The virus did not reach Vanuatu and Samoa, and few cases occurred in Fiji. The collapse of tourism, on land and from cruise ships, resulted in increased unemployment and the closure of hotels and tourism-oriented businesses with multiplier effects throughout the island economies. Many people returned to home islands, putting pressure on local land resources. Diverse local markets, exchange and bartering increased. Women were most affected in terms of lost jobs, more domestic burdens and a rise in domestic violence. This article argues that tourism is unlikely to restart in the immediate future, but may be initiated through small elite ventures. In response, regional metropolitan states – Australia and New Zealand – have increased aid to what is increasingly a strategically important region.

Introduction

In every ocean and sea tourism – increasingly the basis of the economies of most small islands and island states – has been particularly devastated by COVID-19. The virus has had a massive impact on the economies of small island developing states (SIDS) for a range of reasons relating to production, trade and transport, and no economic sector has been more affected than tourism. This article examines the changes that have occurred as a result of the coronavirus shock in three island states that have been particularly affected, almost entirely indirectly because of border closures, and examines the dynamic social, economic and international political implications of these developments.

The SIDS most affected by the collapse of tourism have all been in the Pacific, because of the loss of transport connections with source countries, despite COVID-19 having had minimal direct local impact. This paper focuses on the three SIDS – Samoa, Fiji and Vanuatu – where tourism had been steadily growing during the twenty-first century and where it had become a cornerstone of the economy. In each case, these economies have undergone massive contractions, as much as 20% for Fiji, all unprecedented since independence, with the coronavirus having a much greater economic than health impact. Broadly what has proved true of these states is true of other Pacific SIDS, such as Palau and Tonga, where tourism was also of significance.

In Vanuatu, Fiji and Samoa the impacts of the virus followed in the wake of Cyclone Harold (that had just devastated the northern islands of Vanuatu) and a severe measles epidemic that had taken more than 80 lives in Samoa in 2019 (which severely reduced tourism numbers). Since the measles epidemic had originated in migration from New Zealand that at least offered a warning on how to defend against the pandemic. In Vanuatu, emergency relief was complicated by the need for physical distancing and other regulations as assistance came from overseas. The island economies were thus not in great shape, alongside structural weaknesses, further complicated in Vanuatu by a national election in March that resulted in a change of government.

The challenging context

Despite the rapid spread of COVID-19 elsewhere, because of very limited physical international contact – almost entirely by shipping (and a handful of humanitarian flights) Samoa and Vanuatu have been almost entirely without COVID-19. At the end of October 2020, Fiji, with many more connections with other countries, had had just 33 cases and two deaths. Despite these low numbers, their 'highly tourist-dependent economies' (as they were classified by the Asian Development Bank) were devastated by the border closures, in place by the end of March 2020. That affected both land-based tourism (mainly in resorts) and hitherto fast-growing cruise tourism. The collapse of tourism resulted in a range of both simple and complex repercussions and outcomes, leading to an economic crisis with social and political overtones, in a region of increased strategic significance. However, the early closure of borders prevented the spread of the virus to most SIDS, unlike its more rapid spread, with long-term consequences, in dependent territories in the Pacific, notably Guam and, to a lesser extent, French Polynesia, where international routes were not immediately cut.

Until the COVID-19 pandemic, tourism was increasingly the backbone of the island economies, and particularly dominant in Fiji. With a population of around 950,000, Fiji claimed as many as 100,000 workers employed directly and indirectly in the tourism industry (about 45% of the labour force) serving almost 900,000 visitors in 2019. The industry contributed about 40% of GDP. Samoa and Vanuatu had smaller industries with around 135.000 and 300,000 tourists, respectively. As in Fiji, these industries were slowly growing, with each country diversifying its main sources of tourists from traditional Australia and New Zealand to China and elsewhere. Tourism represented the single most important component of GDP and of the wage and salary labour force, and in each of the countries was a particularly valuable source of foreign exchange. The absolute and immediate loss of such a valuable industry was unprecedented.

While borders were never entirely closed – as humanitarian flights, fishing fleets, occasional cargo ships and yachts brought arrivals of various kinds – the impact was dramatic. Formal statistics are starkly revealing. In the April–June quarter, Fiji officially earned F$4.2 million from tourism, compared with F$528.8 million the previous year. That came from less than a thousand visitors, just four of whom declared themselves to be on holiday; most were ships' crew. In September 2020, Fiji welcomed 1005 visitors for the month compared with 81,354 in the previous September (Radio New Zealand, 30 September 2020). Vanuatu and Samoa, not being regional centres like Fiji, had a tiny fraction of that mobility, and no more tourists. Effectively the SIDS were isolated and cut off from the rest of the world.

Impacts

The immediate and highly visible outcome of the virus was the effective closure of much of the tourist economy: initially of hotels and resorts (although they retained skeleton staff for maintenance and security), followed by businesses oriented to tourism (such as dive shops and tour operators), and a massive downturn in the business of activities that significantly catered to tourists (such as restaurants, bars, hire cars, golf courses, handicraft manufacture and taxis, but also port and airport workers, and many small stores and market operators). Typically the owner of an upmarket resort in Vanuatu – The Havannah – 'had to pause all our community engagement activities which include sourcing supplies from locally based market providers, handicraft producers, local tour operators and the nearby village businesses (for transport, security, community conservation and handyman services)' (as cited in Naupa, 2020). Beyond them were the more informal workers, ranging from musicians, culture centre workers, and the farmers and fishers who supplied hotel markets. The overall impact was greatest on the urban informal sector, who were more likely to experience consequent poverty. Since tourism is labour-intensive many jobs were lost and more than half of those who lost jobs were women working in hotels and restaurants. Multiplier effects were considerable. Without incomes, consumer spending declined as households could no longer support stores and markets and unemployment soared, adding, in each country, to already high youth unemployment. Closures were sudden and unexpected and urban workers had no opportunity to establish alternative livelihoods, even where that was feasible.

In each of the SIDS an immediate response of the hotel industry lay in attempts to stimulate domestic tourism, which had hitherto been of minimal significance, to keep hotels functional and justify some retention of staff, especially skilled workers (such as accountants and chefs). Hotels and resorts – especially those near the capital cities – offered special packages with reduced rates, held special dinner functions, offered to host conferences and provided cheap lunches. This was most successful in Fiji, centred on a 'Love our Locals Fiji' campaign, because of the relatively larger concentration of well-paid salaried workers in the capital, Suva, some frustrated at their inability to travel further.

Most resorts laid off at least half their staff and some quite quickly shut down entirely. The collapse was rapid. Some larger resorts retained workers to take advantage of empty facilities by engaging in more comprehensive maintenance and environmental management (such as mangrove planting) that might offer long-term benefits. By May 2020, barely 3 month after border closure, 50% of tourism businesses in Fiji had closed down or were 'hibernating' (with no ongoing activity), and 35% were functioning but with a reduced workforce, and it was anticipated that 29% of all the tourism businesses would have become bankrupt within 6 months (Wainiqolo, 2020). The firms that were most likely to close down were small and medium-sized locally owned activities without international linkages.

Each of the three states introduced some limited forms of fiscal stimulus package, welfare provision and social cash transfers, as in Samoa directed primarily at former workers in the tourism industry, but these did not extend far, rarely extended to the informal sector or met the needs of the very poor. The SIDS had to borrow internationally to support welfare packages, a process that could not be sustained. Food banks were valuable in Fiji, and NGOs such as Foundation for Rural Integrated Enterprises and Development (FRIEND) provided staple food packages. In Samoa, some hotels did the same for their now redundant employees.

Core tourism facilities, and the larger resorts, are centred on and around urban areas and hence mainly employed urban workers. Especially in Fiji some of these workers lacked access to land; hence, they had no ongoing agricultural activities to fall back on and develop after jobs were lost. The costs were particularly severe in western Viti Levu, the main island of Fiji, where tourism is concentrated (on the Coral Coast and the two main small island groups), bringing social problems and very significant urban-rural return migration. That was accentuated by similar return migration from urban settlements as informal sector jobs dried up. As the Chief Executive of the Fiji Hotel and Tourism Association, Fantasha Lockington, claimed in June: 'We have a little over 100,000 employees who are no longer employed and there isn't anything else that they can turn to except go back to the land that many of these people have access to do sustainable farming for themselves' (as cited in Fox, 2020).

In turn, again especially in Fiji, as many urban jobs were lost, the resultant resurgence of agriculture and fishing transferred problems to rural areas with new pressure on resources and disputes over access and land tenure. Such circumstances were also typical of the Solomon Islands where urban-rural migration was substantial (Eriksson et al., 2020). This contributed to some revaluation of 'tradition' and of subsistence security, especially since international food supply chains became problematic, pushing up the prices of imported food. This offered early indications of improved nutrition as local production and consumption increased, notably in Vanuatu, but less so in Fiji, where urban households especially were more likely to be food-short. Urban gardening was ultimately inadequate for local needs. Again the urban poor were the most affected, because of movement restrictions, lack of access to land elsewhere and increased commodity prices (Davila & Wilkes, 2020). Vanuatu, with a more 'traditional' economy, was thus better placed to survive the economic slump than more 'modernised' Samoa and Fiji. where more employment was in the formal sector.

A further outcome was a profusion of roadside stalls in each of the countries as households tried to generate income from agricultural surpluses and fishing. Since many households sought to sell similar goods, and money was in short supply, in Fiji and Samoa particularly there was revitalisation of more traditional exchange relationships and a revival of bartering. In Fiji, beyond more common exchanges of fish and taro, pigs could be swapped for roofing iron, baked goods for children's toys and food for tutoring of children unable to attend school because of COVID-19 restrictions. As many of 165,000 people joined a Facebook group, 'Barter for Better Fiji', while smaller group catered for specific towns, with a similar group and pattern emerging in Samoa (Boodoosingh, 2020; Darmadi, 2020). Flea markets emerged, especially in Fijian towns, as an urban parallel. While benefits came from the profusion of urban and rural markets previously established long-term vendors now faced strong competition and suffered reduced sales.

Contributing to the problem of lost income support was a decline in remittances – a massive source of income in both Fiji (where it was now more valuable than the sugar industry) and Samoa, and which had been growing rapidly in Vanuatu, with access to New Zealand and Australia under the Recognised Seasonal Employer and Seasonal Worker Program schemes. The latter also ended abruptly when air transport closed down. The absence of COVID-19 in the Northern Territory (Australia), and pressure from mango growers there, resulted in two plane loads of more than 300 workers arriving from Vanuatu in October, as the seasonal worker scheme restarted experimentally. By

November the scheme was being extended further with more arrivals from Fiji and Solomon Islands. In Samoa, as in other SIDS, remittances ordinarily from long-term migrants grew rapidly after hazards (Le De et al., 2014) but parallel economic decline in the source countries – especially New Zealand – meant that long-term and short-term migrants were experiencing unemployment and income stress and were no longer in a position to respond. While the World Bank had estimated a 20% downturn in receipts over the first three months of 2020 the decline was not as great as anticipated, but growth in receipts fell only slightly in Fiji and Samoa, declining more in Vanuatu.

Domestic violence increased as more people experienced frustrating circumstances, such as unemployment, and were 'stuck' at home. NGOs reported significant rises in violence, with the Fiji Women's Crisis Centre receiving more than 500 calls from victims in the first half of the year while the Fiji Ministry of Women recorded 1545 cases of assault against women, with a tenfold increase between March and April. Almost half the women reported a correlation between COVID-19 and violence linked directly to restrictions of movement and strain on families (Radio New Zealand, 24 September 2020). That occurred as many women were experiencing a greater economic and emotional load, and extra home and caring roles, undoing previous gains for women in access to employment. Mental health was also believed to be worsening. Ordinary crime also increased; around Nadi in Fiji, hundreds of incidents of crop theft replaced two or three a week before the crisis. That prompted Shamima Ali, the Director of the Fiji Women's Crisis Centre, to argue that although Fijians might be resilient 'we must stop romanticizing the Fijian way of life, the traditional mechanisms' since not everyone had land and rural homes to return to (as cited in Doherty, 2020). In Vanuatu, too theft of kava plants, sandalwood trees and root crops also occurred (Davila & Wilkes, 2020). The complex responses and restructuring that border closures required could not simply be accommodated by return to an older order.

A future tourist industry?

Unlike most other crises, but similar to more localised recent epidemics like Ebola, SARS and MERS, there is no indication of when the crisis may be over. Much depends on the discovery of an effective vaccine and its availability. The present crisis in the Pacific SIDS is likely to be sustained for many months, with severe implications for poverty. Based on International Air Transport Association (IATA) expectations on the challenges to airline regeneration and restructuring, after their parallel collapse, by mid-2020 it was already feared that the Pacific tourism industry would not return to pre-COVID levels until 2023 (Wainiqolo, 2020), since most Pacific tourists arrive by air and restoring connectivity would be difficult.

While Fiji has a relatively sophisticated health-care system (that has coped reasonably well with its few cases), the SIDS are conscious of the risk that is posed by welcoming visitors to virus-free islands. Despite decades of investment and capacity-building, health systems in the Pacific remain weak, and urban areas have many large households living at high densities with limited services, including clean water. Inevitably the simultaneous loss of so many jobs and the resultant social problems encouraged the desire to re-establish tourism. The Fiji Prime Minister stated in June, 3 months into the crisis: 'By slowly and safely bringing back vital tourism revenue to Fiji we will be in fact saving lives. The long-term cost of complete closures and unemployment would risk doing immense harm to Fijians' mental and physical health' (as cited in Fox, 2020). Getting that balance right, in a dominantly international industry, is a huge challenge. Indeed, much of the tourist infrastructure, from the hotels and resorts, to airlines and hire cars, is owned or franchised by foreign corporations who make key investment decisions elsewhere.

Since the two main sources of tourism in the Pacific SIDS – Australia and New Zealand – were largely free of COVID (with almost all cases coming from overseas), island states hope and anticipate that a travel 'bubble' (air-bridge or airline corridor), slowly opening between New Zealand and Australia, will eventually extend to the Pacific, probably first to the Cook Islands, and enable tourism to resume. Conscious of the circumstances in French Polynesia where borders with the United States and France had been lifted too soon and tourists allowed in, resulting in an unprecedented spike in cases, in October Fiji was anticipating that its borders would remain closed to commercial aircraft until at least March 2021. Nonetheless, Fiji was contemplating a more personalised 'bula bubble' where elite hotels might welcome affluent guests on private aircraft:

> The Laucala Private Island Resort has partnered with Fiji Airways, the country's national airline, enabling up to 20 guests to fly on a private chartered Fiji Airways jet from Los Angeles to Nadi, Fiji's primary airport and main transit hub. From there, they will be transferred to Laucala, where they will have the private island resort all to themselves. Because of Laucala's remoteness the Department of Health has permitted the program to go forward without guests having to isolate for two weeks. They will need three negative Covid-19 tests, though – one two weeks before traveling, one 72 hours before boarding (which will be sent to the tourism authority in order to confirm travel permits) and one upon arrival in Fiji. The cost? A cool 490,000 USD covers the jet, a minimum seven-night stay, on-island activities, food and drink and airport transfers for up to 20 people. (CNN, 2020)

It was not apparent that significant demand existed, yet other resorts in Fiji may develop similar strategies. The Prime Minister had earlier been happy to welcome elite travellers stating:

> So, say you're a billionaire looking to fly your own jet, rent your own island, and invest millions of dollars in Fiji in the process – if you've taken all the necessary health precautions and borne all associated costs, you may have a new home to escape the pandemic in paradise. (quoted in Sullivan, 2020)

A 'blue lane' was created to permit travellers to come to the country via private yacht, with visitors able to serve out their quarantine on board before coming ashore. Vanuatu and Samoa, without elite resorts on their own islands, are unlikely to develop such strategies, while an elite-led recovery of small isolated resorts and small cruises can only have limited impact on economic development and employment, with minimal trickledown effect since most expenditure occurs outside the SIDS.

The future of cruise ships, quickly dismissed by many as 'floating petri dishes', and increasingly perceived as presenting problems of air and marine pollution is as uncertain. Cruise ships will seek to follow suit and return, again with a focus on small islands such as the Mamanuca and Yasawa Islands (Fiji), and with smaller, elite cruise ships with fewer than a hundred passengers. Despite the health hazards attached to cruise ships, and the future challenges in their avoiding capital cities, they had previously been attractive in most Pacific SIDS since their cruise itineraries included outlying islands where tourism and economic development were otherwise limited.

Planning quickly began in anticipation of the industry reopening. Chris Cocker, the CEO of the Pacific Tourism Organisation (SPTO), suggested: 'We are going to move towards most likely green tourism and sustainable tourism because we have seen the oneness that COVID-19, in a positive way, has done to our environment. I think the importance of sustainable tourism will increase as we move towards recovering and moving forward for the future of tourism in the Pacific, and the world as a whole' (Radio New Zealand, 12 May 2020). A quickly produced Vanuatu *Tourism Crises Response and Recovery Plan* draft of May pointed out:

> Our tourism industry has been developed in a way that has undermined our subsistence capacities which has made some communities and households dependent and vulnerable. With the absence of formal safety nets in Vanuatu, informal community and culturally based social protection systems (brought about through the traditional economy) are more vital than ever before (Vanuatu Department of Tourism, 2020, p. 4)

This idealistic plan sought to move away from 'business as usual', promote local linkages (from agriculture to soap manufacture), smaller-scale tourism and local values. Former tourism workers may have their own distinctive approach to future employment in the industry. As some Fijian displaced workers were reported: 'People are saying, yes, we will have to return to our jobs, because we need the money to pay for our bills, school fees etcetera, but at the same time they are reflecting on how this should be done, with one particular group of respondents saying that tourism must complement their way of life and not overtake everything else' (Radio New Zealand, 26 October 2020). More than a third of Fijian tourism workers were wary about staying in the industry and contemplated the possibility of better jobs in creative industries (Movono & Scheyvens, 2020).

However, by the time that the Vanuatu Tourism Crisis Response and Recovery Plan emerged in October 2020 (Vanuatu Department of Tourism, 2020), it had lost its sustainable edge and established 'five pillars' in the most general terms: safeguarding the health of citizens and visitors; planning for moving people internationally and nationally in a COVID environment; ensuring tourism businesses are financially viable and ready to launch their products again when the time is right; helping to build international demand for Vanuatu tourism, including through messaging that Vanuatu wants to be part of the proposed New Zealand and Australia tourism bubble and finally ensuring good communications throughout Vanuatu about the changes taking place within the sector. None of this was particularly new. Likewise, the SPTO's own Pacific Tourism recovery plan of June (Forward, 2020) was little more than a conventional business development report. Samoa and Fiji had yet to suggest any change in long-term strategies. Within such an important industry intense competition for an emergent market may become significant and challenge the widespread notion in tourism (and other economic and social arenas) that a 'new normal' will be necessary and somehow emerge. Large resorts may be seen by tourists as self-contained and secure from any possible local viruses and by local people as sites to contain visitors from countries with recent COVID-19 clusters.

Ultimately, the future of tourism is even more uncertain than the end of the coronavirus crisis. As the crisis remains in place, the infrastructure of the industry – airlines (particularly regional airlines), international resorts, travel agents and cruise ships – may simply fold as debts mount. So too supply chains. Collapse of airlines may render some destinations inaccessible. Future fare structures are unpredictable. A 'bubble' enabling tourism from New Zealand and Australia would avoid SIDS falling into a poverty and debt trap, creating insecurity and so drawing on overseas aid, but a bubble is not imminent. Staycations may be more attractive and are being encouraged in key markets such as Australia and New Zealand. Small elite cruises and flights with well-off passengers are most likely to be the first to revive. Ironically the high-end resorts with least direct economic linkage to the islands, such as Laucala and Turtle Cove, in Fiji – may prove to be the survivors (since their owners are less likely to go under and they provide isolated cocoons). That may be a boost for conservation: a tiny silver lining in ravaged economies. While island scale precludes substantial diversity, the ongoing experience of COVID-19 provides a harsh lesson that some greater diversity and self-reliance are essential. Desperation to revive may produce a 'new normal' much like the old rather than a more ambitious 'green', sustainable, cultural and regional tourism. Forecasting the future of tourism is now more problematic than ever, and a vaccine may reshape all contemporary conjectures.

Conclusion

For economies so focused on tourism, the immediate future is bleak. The collapse of the industry in the Pacific has given rise to significant gender and poverty implications, since women particularly lost jobs in the service industries and experienced the rise in domestic violence, a pattern earlier occurring in countries experiencing other pandemics (Wenham et al., 2020) and consistent with the outcomes of other less significant shocks (Donahue et al., 2014). Moreover, the businesses that have been most likely to close down were locally owned: a real blow to national small business. As many as a third of households in each of these SIDS lived below poverty lines of US$5.50 per day prior to the crisis (Hoy, 2020), and more are likely to have now been pushed into extreme poverty. After unprecedented economic losses, experienced in partial isolation, and with most countries focused on national concerns, it will be difficult to regain the confidence and the connections to rebuild. The benefits of regional cooperation will be challenged as all SIDS pursue tourism within an uncertain market.

While tourist numbers have bounced back quickly after cyclones, and the prospect of visiting nearby islands that have not experienced the virus is attractive to tourists from the main sources of Australia and New Zealand, this is a new era. However, despite possible concerns over health-care systems, destination images of the islands as clean and green and disease free can only be helpful. The present relative isolation may be turned into an advantage. But that will necessarily mean that the SIDS will need to ensure they have adequate health-care systems in place.

COVID-19 offers a new and pointed focus on the basic challenges to economic development in SIDS – where resources are limited, opportunities for diversification are restricted and the subsistence base has been eroded. In each of the Pacific SIDS, some return to rural life has occurred, along with the revival of past practices of exchange and bartering. Remarkably similar return migration and revival of bartering have occurred in islands elsewhere, from the Solomon Islands to Bali (Laula & Paddock, 2020). Mobility is a key part of resilience. That may ensure a greater respect for tradition and a determination to retain a strong subsistence base, and this reversal and partial revival of local foods may strengthen the quest for food security and more adequate nutrition (Farrell et al., 2020). Equally, pressure for national incomes might result in a rush back to the old order rather than using the crisis as a window of opportunity for seeking to build back better.

Until tourism regains strength, remittances will be invaluable and islander residents in New Zealand and Australia will come under-renewed pressure to support kin at home. Thousands of Pacific workers in each of the Pacific SIDS have been unable to go to New Zealand and Australia under the seasonal worker schemes because of pandemic travel restriction. They, and many others, will return as soon as it is viable. Samoa and Vanuatu especially have engaged in negotiations to try and increase participant numbers and bring forward a safe and extended implementation. Several Pacific SIDS are anxious that the Australia's Pacific Labour Scheme (a new extension of the seasonal scheme, that offers employment in other sectors, including hospitality and caring, and for longer periods of time) also be stepped up to enable more islanders to gain incomes in Australia. Labour migration, and other forms of migration, will be more vital.

COVID-19 has emphasised the geopolitical significance of the Pacific region. Australia and New Zealand have recently claimed a 'Pacific step-up' and a 'Pacific reset', respectively, marking intendedly closer engagement with the region, to offset China's growing presence, and its concessional loans, and ensure increased aid delivery (where, especially for Australia, the national climate change policy was anathema in the region where it was seen as inaction). By October Australia had pledged an additional US$500 in aid for the region to roll out a regional immunisation programme. That was quickly dubbed 'vaccine diplomacy' in response to Chinese 'mask diplomacy' since China had quickly delivered masks and other protective equipment. The Pacific SIDS need significant aid (complicated by the Chinese presence in a strategically significant region) and it is crucial to the traditional aid donors – Australia and New Zealand – that 'failed states' do not emerge in the region. Thus in the last 2 years, neither country welcomed the prospect of either an independent Bougainville, despite overwhelming island support for its secession from Papua New Guinea, or an independent New Caledonia. Yet aid resources may be scarce as metropolitan states face rising levels of debt and seek to rebuild their own economies. Moreover, the COVID-19 crisis is seen as a forerunner of a potentially greater crisis: climate change. The Secretary General of the Pacific Island Forum, Meg Taylor, has stated: 'The COVID-19 public health emergency and its ensuing humanitarian and economic fallout offers us a glimpse of what the global climate emergency can become if it is left unchecked and if we do not act now' (as cited in McAdam & Pryke, 2020). COVID-19 will lead to new relationships in this strategic arena, rather more than changes in the structure of tourism, that will be just one part of a restructuring of political and economic systems as part of an inevitably uncertain 'new normal'.

Disclosure statement

No potential conflict of interest was reported by the author.

References

Boodoosingh, R. (2020, June 30). Bartering in Samoa during COVID-19. *ANU DevPolicyBlog*.
CNN. (2020, October 30). Fiji resort offers the ultimate in social distancing. *CNN*.

Darmadi, G. (2020, June 1). Fijians turn to bartering system as coronavirus shutdowns cause mass unemployment. *ABC News.*

Davila, F., & Wilkes, B. (2020). *COVID-19 and food systems in Pacific island countries, in ACIAR, COVID-19 and food states in the Indo-Pacific: An assessment of vulnerabilities, impacts and opportunities for action.* ACIAR Technical Report No 96 (pp. 94–126). ACIAR.

Doherty, B. (2020, June 29). Quarter of businesses in Pacific fear they will not survive Covid-19 pandemic. *Guardian.*

Donahue, J., Eccles, K., & Miller-Dawkins, M. (2014). Responding to shocks: Women's experiences of economic shocks in the Solomon Islands and Vanuatu. In S. Feeny (Ed.), *Household vulnerability and resilience to economic shocks: Findings from Melanesia* (pp. 43–66). Routledge.

Eriksson, H., Ride, A., Boso, D., Sukul, M., Batalofo, M., Siota, F., & Gomese, C. (2020). *Changes and adaptations in village food systems in Solomon Islands. A rapid appraisal during the early stages of the COVID-19 pandemic.* WorldFish Program Report No 2020:20. WorldFish.

Farrell, P., Thow, A.-M., Wate, J., Nonga, N., Vatucawaqa, P., Brewer, T., Sharp, M. K., Farmery, A., Trevena, H., Reeve, E., Eriksson, H., Gonzalez, I., Mulcahy, G., Eurich, J. G., & Andrew, N. L. (2020). COVID-19 and Pacific food system resilience: Opportunities to build a robust response. *Food Security, 12*(4), 783–791. https://doi.org/10.1007/s12571-020-01087-y

Forward. (2020). *Pacific tourism: COVID-19 impact and recovery. Scenario development and recovery pathways.* SPTO.

Fox, L. (2020, June 25). Fiji proposes a 'Bula Bubble' to allow Australians to travel during the coronavirus pandemic. *ABC News.*

Hoy, C. (2020, July 33-37). Poverty and the pandemic in the Pacific. *Pacific Economic Monitor.*

Laula, N., & Paddock, R. (2020, July 20). With tourists gone, Bali workers return to farms and fishing. *New York Times.*

Le De, L., Gaillard, J.-C., Friesen, W., & Smith, F. (2014). Remittances in the face of disasters: A case study of rural Samoa. *Environment, Development and Sustainability, 17*(3), 653–672. https://doi.org/10.1007/s10668-014-9559-0

McAdam, J., & Pryke, J. (2020, October 27). Preparing for when climate change drives people from their homes. *The Interpreter.*

Movono, A., & Scheyvens, R. (2020, November 25). Pacific tourism is desperate for a vaccine and travel freedoms, but the industry must learn from this crisis. *The Conversation.*

Naupa, A. (2020, July 29). A tale of two sectors: Women leaders bridging the formal and informal sectors during Vanuatu's COVID crisis. *PacNews.*

Sullivan, R. (2020, June 28). Fiji markets itself as retreat for billionaires during pandemic. *CNN.*

Vanuatu Department of Tourism. (2020). *The VSTP tourism crises response and recovery plan (2020-2023).*

Wainiqolo, I. (2020, July 7-8). COVID-19 and the Fiji economy: An opportunity to reorient public spending. *Pacific Economic Monitor.*

Wenham, C., Smith, J., Davies, S., Feng, H., Grépin, K. A., Harman, S., Herten-Crabb, A., & Morgan, R. (2020, July). Women are most affected by pandemics – Lessons from past outbreaks. *Nature, 583*(7815), 194–198. https://doi.org/10.1038/d41586-020-02006-z

OPEN ACCESS

COVID-19 and the British Overseas Territories: a comparative view

Matthew C. Benwell, Peter Clegg and Alasdair Pinkerton

ABSTRACT

The British Overseas Territories are part of the 'Commonwealth family', and have characteristics such as isolation, economic vulnerability, and small populations, which have influenced how the territories have tackled COVID-19. Their direct relationship with Britain has been another important consideration. The article focuses on four of the Overseas Territories – the Falkland Islands, Gibraltar, British Virgin Islands, and Pitcairn – and considers their responses to, and challenges caused by, the pandemic. Overall, the territories have effectively managed the initial period of the pandemic, but each is under significant strain and in some instances the relationship with Britain has become more difficult. Indeed, COVID has exacerbated pre-existing tensions between the territories and London.

Introduction

Though not members of the Commonwealth of Nations *per se*, Britain's 14 Overseas Territories (BOTs) are part of the broader 'Commonwealth family', and are particularly interesting places to study within the context of COVID-19. Many of the BOTs are defined by their relative isolation, vulnerability, small populations, and value as geo-strategic sites for the projection of military power. Unlike the independent members of the Commonwealth, the territories all have direct constitutional, political and economic links to Britain, and rely on it for their defence and foreign affairs. This liminality – being neither independent sovereign nations nor constituent parts of Britain – is a long-standing source of debate and contestation, and has been brought into starker relief during the pandemic.

Several issues animate the contemporary relationship between the OTs and Britain, including the economic and security-related challenges posed by Brexit (Benwell & Pinkerton, 2016; Clegg, 2016); strained constitutional relations, related *inter alia* to the imposition of anti-money laundering laws and social legislation enhancing LGBTQ+ rights (Yusuf & Chowdhury, 2019); as well as concerns over Britain's responsiveness to aid and reconstruction in the aftermath of natural disasters (see Clegg, 2018; Pinkerton & Benwell, 2017). As recently as September 2020 tensions between the British-appointed

Governor to the British Virgin Islands (BVI) and the territory's Premier risked a constitutional crisis over the Governor's decision to invite the Royal Navy to shore up the territory's maritime borders in response to the COVID-19 pandemic (CNW, 2020). Underlying many of these tensions is the issue of race, with a perception among Caribbean citizens of the OTs that the British government is failing to understand or support the interests and value of them, while privileging other territories such as the Falkland Islands and Gibraltar, and the Crown Dependencies. This supports a view in the Caribbean territories, in particular, that Britain continues to act in a neo-colonial way treating the OTs as junior rather than full partners in ways that make problematic assumptions about their ability to govern and manage their own affairs.

The article focuses on four of the OTs – the Falkland Islands, Gibraltar, BVI, and Pitcairn – and considers their responses to, and challenges caused by, the pandemic. The territories were chosen because of their divergent geographical locations in the South Atlantic, Mediterranean, Caribbean and southern Pacific Ocean respectively that have caused specific challenges. In addition, the four reflect different economic and social conditions, e.g., in regard to local budgetary strength, key economic sectors, and population and demographic concerns. They are also representative of the challenges being faced across the territories. Further, the selection of the four foregrounds several significant over-arching themes that thread through the case studies that include: the domestic responses of the respective BOT governments and how these worked alongside, and sometimes came into conflict with, the financial, diplomatic and logistical support provided by the British government; the sense of precarity experienced in the BOTs as a result of their geographical isolation *or* anxieties over the policing of borders; concerns about economic insecurities; and the opportunities the pandemic presented to the BOTs to demonstrate their sovereign capacity. Our analysis begins with the Falkland Islands.

Falkland Islands

The first case of COVID-19 was confirmed in the Falkland Islands on 3 April 2020. The patient was a British serviceperson stationed at RAF Mount Pleasant who was later transferred from the military base to the only civilian hospital on the islands, the King Edward Memorial Hospital. A health team commenced contact tracing and in the following weeks of April a total of 13 cases of COVID-19 were diagnosed. All the cases stemmed from the military base and all patients recovered (Falkland Islands Government, 2020). While several members of the civilian population in the Falklands went into self-isolation with symptoms, no cases of COVID-19 were seen initially outside of Mount Pleasant. However, in mid-November, two cases in the general population were reported (Penguin News, 2020). The threat posed to the 3000-strong civilian population of the Falkland Islands by COVID-19 is particularly serious given that about 'a sixth of the population is classed as high-risk, mainly those over 70 with underlying health conditions' (Haynes, 2020). The Falkland Islands Government (FIG) and medical staff were acutely aware of the potential impacts an outbreak could have and prepared accordingly, reorganising hospital and staffing arrangements at the hospital, as well as ensuring they had adequate supplies of medical equipment and pharmaceuticals. Members of the Falkland Islands' community were also praised by the Governor, Nigel Phillips, for their resourcefulness and voluntary work during the pandemic (MercoPress, 2020a).

The relative isolation of the Falkland Islands in the South-West Atlantic was a double-edged sword during the early months of the pandemic. On the one hand, it ensured that the Falklands remained well behind the high rates of infection witnessed in other parts of the world, including Britain. The FIG enforced strict quarantine measures on those arriving in the islands and flights between South America (Brazil and Chile, both of which experienced serious outbreaks of COVID-19) and the Falklands were cut in early April with these disruptions to airlinks set to continue into 2021 (MercoPress, 2020c). Yet, on the other hand, this isolation is a stark reminder of the precarity of life in the islands. With no flights operating to South America (aside from a repatriation flight to Punta Arenas, Chile, in late July) the only airlink to the outside world was with Britain, some 8,000 miles away. This created considerable inconvenience, especially for citizens from South American countries living in the islands. Also, in March 2020, flights between Britain and the Falklands were disrupted, 'as border closures around the world left the defence ministry planes with nowhere to stop to refuel on the long journey. That meant the Falklands were unable to send coronavirus tests to labs in the UK. It also left a group of around 20 high schoolers, who were in the UK for their final years of secondary education, stranded away from their families' (Roberts, as cited in Nugent, 2020). In these early stages of the pandemic, then, this isolation brought severe logistical challenges at a critical moment in the global outbreak of COVID-19, as well as more intimate disruptions to families.

Initially, the Falkland Islands had no capacity to conduct tests for COVID-19 meaning samples, once the airlink was re-established, had to be flown back to Britain with results taking roughly 10 days to process. In the second half of May 2020 with the help of the British Government, the Falklands secured equipment to undertake testing without the need to send samples back to Britain. Two intensive treatment units with a small medical team were deployed to the Falklands and the Royal Air Force (RAF) flew in extra supplies of oxygen and medicine (Ministry of Defence, 2020). British military engineers also adapted oxygen units from Tornado and Hercules aircraft for use as hospital-grade, life support units (Foreign & Commonwealth Office, 2020). Conservative MP and chair of the All-Party Parliamentary Group on the BOTs, Andrew Rosindell, had referred to the pandemic as a 'ticking time bomb' for the territories, stating, 'we have a duty, a responsibility, not to forget these places' (McGrath, 2020). These statements preceded the emergency logistical responses in the Falklands and elsewhere, and were a timely reminder to the British Government of its commitments to the OTs in times of crisis. However, and as we consider later in relation to the BVI, the British response has been criticised for not recognising local needs and sensibilities. Concerns that have been amplified by alleged past failures and heavy handedness in relation to Britain's response to the impact of Hurricane Irma in the BVI and Anguilla, and the political, economic and security fallout from Brexit, of which Rosindell was a supporter (Benwell & Pinkerton, 2016; Byron, 2019; Clegg, 2018; Pinkerton & Benwell, 2017).

Finally, the pandemic brought to the fore some of the long-running economic and geopolitical insecurities facing the Falkland Islands. The islands' economy, with its heavy reliance on fisheries, agriculture and tourism, is particularly susceptible to global market shocks resulting in an uncertain short-term future. The Executive Secretary of the Falkland Islands Fishing Companies Association, James Bates, stated that, 'COVID-19 is of course a major challenge but in addition the consequences of Brexit are still unknown but potentially damaging. Also, recent increases in costs, and the political rhetoric from Argentina and their efforts to obstruct our development have become increasingly menacing' (MercoPress, 2020b). Both concerns have been heightened after the Falklands (and the other OTs) were excluded from the UK-EU trade deal signed on 30 December 2020. The pandemic has coincided with growing diplomatic pressure from Argentina in their sovereignty dispute with Britain that has understandably not been well received in the Falklands (offers of humanitarian assistance from Buenos Aires received no response from the FIG). Indeed, the epidemiological claiming of cases of COVID-19 in the Falklands by Argentina for inclusion in its national statistics (Télam, 2020), is a troubling reminder of the unrelenting sovereignty aspirations of their near and threatening neighbour.

Gibraltar

In the nine months since recording its first confirmed case on 3 March 2020, Gibraltar reported 943 coronavirus cases (to 19 November), with 742 confirmed recoveries and three deaths (HM Government of Gibraltar, 2020a). Coronavirus' arrival in Gibraltar was attributed to a young couple returning to Gibraltar from northern Italy via Malaga Airport in southern Spain, one of whom subsequently developed symptoms and self-isolated until he had recovered. A precautionary test confirmed COVID-19 and the Gibraltar Heath Authority was reported to have started the process of identifying all healthcare workers with whom the young man had been in contact, as well as launching an 'extensive process of contact tracing' (Dollimore, 2020). This seemed to be a successful first deployment of public health procedures designed to prevent and/or identify the spread of COVID-19 through the territory's 34,000 population. However, since late August cases have grown quickly. In response, Chief Minister Fabian Picardo argued that Gibraltar was being judged unfairly over the rise in cases. He said that 'If you do a more detailed dive and you look at the fact that we are doing more testing than most places per head of population, then you'll understand that we are now being very successful at identifying cases of the virus and then exercising controls in terms of imposing self-isolation, etc.' (Calder, 2020). This argument has helped persuade the British Government to retain Gibraltar on its travel corridor list of countries, territories and regions (alongside every other BOT) (Department of Transport, 2021)

The institutional connections between the Gibraltar Health Authority and the National Health Service in Britain contributed to a close mirroring of the public health response to COVID-19 in both countries, albeit with contingencies timed to respond to the particular epidemiological profile of the territory. The increase in ventilator capacity, from five at the emergence of the pandemic to 50 in late March, was judged a triumph of procurement (Cavilla, 2020). Serendipitously, Gibraltar's newly-completed oxygen production plant (commissioned to enable the territory's self-sufficiency in medical oxygen after Brexit) was used immediately (Smith, 2020). COVID-19 testing, initially only available via Britain, was by mid-May being undertaken in two new laboratory facilities. With these in place, Gibraltar had the capacity to test two percent of the national population each day, and some speculated that Gibraltar might even be the 'first country to do Covid-19 antibody tests on [the] entire population' (Thomas, 2020). If these achievements were expressions of Gibraltar's scientific and public health competencies (and growing self-sufficiency), the importance of the continuing relationship with Britain was seen with the Ministry of Defence's involvement in constructing a makeshift

'Nightingale Hospital' within the Europa Point Sports Centre, previously the main venue for the International Island Games in July 2020 (GBC, 2020).

Unlike BOTs that are isolated islands (Pitcairn, the Falkland Islands, and St Helena to name but a few), Gibraltar has a highly porous land border with Spain. On any given working day somewhere between ten and twenty thousand people cross the frontier – the vast majority travelling into Gibraltar in the morning for paid employment or for tourism, with a reverse flow in the evening as those same workers and tourists return home to their accommodation inside Spain. This is a daily migration that sustains communities and economies on either side of the border and is generally considered to be symbiotic and mutually beneficial, although it is important to note that the border was closed altogether in 1967 under General Franco, only reopening in 1986 and is still subject to occasional politically-motivated 'delays'. When, in late-March and April, Spain was confirmed as a global hot spot of COVID-19 infections, the frontier became a particular focal point of anxiety for public health practitioners in Gibraltar (ITV News, 2020).

Somewhat defying historical precedent, the frontier has not become a site of geopolitical tension during the course of the pandemic so far, in fact quite the opposite. The Gibraltarian and Spanish governments have worked closely and collaboratively to ensure that border-dependent communities in Gibraltar and southern Spain have been minimally inconvenienced by COVID-19 contingencies and international travel restrictions. Gibraltar's Chief Minister, Picardo, revealed in a tweet that Spain and Gibraltar were 'working together' and 'keeping border fluidity whilst respecting the State of Emergency in Spain and restrictions in #Gibraltar' (Picardo, 2020). Even during the tightest periods of lockdown, the frontier remained open for anyone with a work contract to cross, although Gibraltar's hotels (empty through loss of tourism) helped minimise border crossings by providing accommodation to construction workers, while the University of Gibraltar's halls of residence were opened up to non-resident healthcare professionals (Montegriffo, 2020). The Government of Gibraltar's *Unlock the Rock* (2020) plan for post-lockdown recovery (published in May 2020) offers an important insight into the particular challenges of balancing pandemic- and geopolitical- risk in a precarious environment such as Gibraltar. As the report states, 'The greatest threat to Gibraltar of a return of large numbers of persons infected with COVID-19 will be from arrivals from outside Gibraltar. It is unrealistic, however, to pretend that Gibraltar can operate as an island, without cross-frontier workers or without human arrivals from the UK' (HM Government of Gibraltar, 2020b). A message that has been reinforced by the post-Brexit efforts to keep the border open between Gibraltar and Spain.

British Virgin Islands

The first cases of COVID-19 in the BVI were recorded on 25 March, with several further cases in April and early May, with one death on 19 April. Then from early May to early August there were no further recorded cases; however, in late August and early September there was a spike. The initial efforts to contain the virus were successful. The BVI followed measures taken elsewhere in the Caribbean: control of movement into the country, control of gatherings, and then control of movement within the country (Murphy et al., 2020). Over the summer internal controls were relaxed, but were tightened again for a few weeks in late August when cases rose. The suspected source of the new outbreak was human smuggling between the BVI and the neighbouring US Virgin Islands that was at the time experiencing a second COVID-19 outbreak.

The BVI's response to the pandemic has been shaped by worsening relations with Britain and its Governor. One area of contention was the package of measures to support the economy. The BVI's important tourism industry was particularly hard hit with hotels, yacht charter companies, restaurants and other tourism related industries being impacted with mass layoffs or cuts to salaries (Wheatley, 2020). Early on the opposition called on the Government led by Premier Andrew Fahie to enact a comprehensive economic stimulus package but it was delayed until the end of May (Ahmed, 2020b). An important reason for the delay was a dispute between the Government and Governor Gus Jaspert over the so called 'Protocols for Effective Financial Management', which had been agreed in 2012. The protocols have been long a source of dispute in the BVI and in other Caribbean BOTs, which limit the amount of borrowing governments can undertake, and if the limit is breached Britain can increase its control of the territories' financial affairs. Fahie argued that the protocols were 'overly restrictive', and were delaying the government's economic response to the crisis; Jaspert responded by defending the protocols saying the government had 'considerable headroom' (Ahmed, 2020a). Later, he stated, 'I have not seen any evidence to indicate that [the Protocols] hamper the government's ability to bring forward an economic package for the people' (Kampa, 2020). Nevertheless, the government was concerned about its limited room for manoeuvre. As was argued, 'the government cannot completely deplete its Reserve Fund of about US$80 million, some of which must be retained for contingencies ... It is also not prudent for the government to pursue a level of borrowing and financial support from the Social Security Board that would ultimately compromise the long-term solvency of the fund' (Wheatley, 2020). It would like Britain to 'demonstrate flexibility on a higher debt threshold for the VI on a permanent basis, particularly given the recent substantial increase in borrowing and debt by governments to rescue their economies from the damage inflicted by the coronavirus, including the UK' (Wheatley, 2020). In 2019 the BVI had a low debt-to-GDP ratio of 18%. When the BVI Government released its stimulus package, which included an unemployment fund; business grants; funds to support the National Health Insurance programme; and allocations for key industries, it also included a cut in the budget for the Governor's Office (The House of Assembly of the Virgin Islands, 2020).

Relations between the BVI Government and the Governor deteriorated further after a falling out over securing the territory's border. The government refused the UK's offer of help to patrol the borders in the early days of the pandemic. But then the Governor overruled Fahie and his ministers, and invited a British Royal Navy vessel, HMS Medway, to help secure the borders using his powers in the BVI Constitution. He defended his position, saying 'As your governor, it is my constitutional responsibility to protect the people of BVI and ensure the security of these islands (CNW, 2020; Waldinger, 2020a). In reply Fahie criticised the decision: 'Yet again, [the] governor has deliberately made public statements that serve to undermine the relationship between the BVI public and their democratically elected government through dangerously misleading misinformation'. He also described the situation as 'the tyranny that is unfolding through Governor Jaspert on behalf of the British Empire' (Waldinger, 2020b). Relations soured further when on 18 January 2021 the Governor instituted an independent judge-led inquiry into allegations of political corruption, misuse of taxpayers' money (including the misappropriation of COVID-relief funds), and a climate of fear in the BVI (Wintour, 2021).

Pitcairn

So far Pitcairn remains free of COVID-19, in large part due to its isolation in the Pacific Ocean. As Filho et al. (2020, p. 3) argued, 'Remoteness, isolation, and inaccessibility have thus far allowed several island states [in the Pacific] to escape infection'. However, the risks are acute. Due to Pitcairn's very small and ageing population, of 40, even one case would pose an existential threat to the community. First detailed discussions of COVID-19 took place on 10 March when the Medical Officer attended the Pitcairn Island Council (PIC) and outlined the nature of the virus and some key measures that the island should take to protect itself (PIC (Pitcairn Island Council), 2020a). One of the first measures was the Council's decision not to allow a cruise ship to land, nor any islanders to board (PIC, 2020b, p. 2). The decision went against the views of many, who in a community questionnaire, suggested that all shipping schedules should continue as normal (PIC, 2020b, p. 1). Soon after the Council decided to ban all short-stay visitors and local traders and officials from boarding vessels (PIC, 2020c).

At the end of March, the Council met again and decided that neither home isolation nor social distancing measures were needed. Also, the meeting discussed who was entitled to travel on the support ship. It was agreed that all permanent Pitcairn residents, essential contracted staff and their partners would be permitted to travel between Pitcairn and New Zealand providing they adhered to all rules and protocols (PIC, 2020d). However, the decision caused disquiet amongst Pitcairners who questioned whether islanders should be allowed to return home during this period. Also, there was discussion about whether non-local contracted staff holding key roles, such as the doctor and teacher, should be sent home (PIC, 2020e, p. 2). The fear (of a very limited number) of outsiders was quite different to the approach taken by Gibraltar.

One important outstanding issue that required a response was what would happen if a Pitcairn resident became ill with COVID-19. It was hoped that a medivac pathway could be established. On 7 April Mayor Charlene Warren-Peu discussed Pitcairn's need for a reliable pathway with Baroness Sugg, the Minister for the BOTs. Subsequently, the British Embassy in Paris advised that French Polynesia responded favourably to the request, and that Pitcairn residents had the right to enter Tahiti; however, this was not a viable option as flights between Mangareva and Tahiti had been suspended (PIC, 2020f). In June it was decided that New Zealand would become Pitcairn's approved medical pathway (PIC, 2020i). Pitcairn's response to COVID-19 was further refined in May. The Medical Officer stated at a Special Council Meeting on 21 May that 'Pitcairn has zero capacity to manage a mild or severe case of the disease. If the virus were to reach Pitcairn, the risk and number of potential deaths has greatly increased [compared to previous information]' (PIC, 2020g, p. 1). The Medical Officer also remarked that Public Health England 'agree that greater emphasis has to go into keeping Pitcairn free of the virus' (PIC, 2020g, p. 2). However, a little later when advice was provided that social distancing measures for residents should again be considered the Island Council declined to give its support (PIC, 2020h, p. 6).

Although Pitcairn receives most of its budget from the British government, COVID-19 is having an impact on the economy, particularly from the loss of cruise ship visitors.

As a consequence, Britain's Department for International Development provided a debt support package for on-island permanent residents, worth NZ$171,000. The Council added a further NZ$4000 from its discretionary fund, which meant each adult resident would receive NZ$555.55 per month until March 2021. However, the Administrator made clear that due to COVID-19 less money would be made available to Pitcairn going forward, and so for instance, the cost of the shipping service would have to be reviewed (PIC, 2020i). COVID has exacerbated both Pitcairn's own vulnerability and the British government's willingness to maintain the same level of financial support as it has previously. The small and ageing population, the extremely narrow economic base, the legacy of child sex abuse convictions, the suspicion of outsiders, and the loss of crucial EU funds as a result of Brexit are putting at risk the territory's viability.

COVID-19 in context

The impact of COVID-19 on the BOTs has come at a difficult time in their relations with Britain, perhaps the most difficult since the late 1990s. Several events and issues have damaged trust and respect. The decision of Britain to leave the EU was significant, as none of the territories were in favour, although of course only Gibraltarians had a vote. The EU provided important benefits to the OTs, including in relation to trade access, bilateral and regional aid, and policy engagement in Brussels (Clegg, 2016). The OTs are not confident that Britain will make good the losses. Then there were criticisms of Britain's response to Hurricane Irma, which badly affected Anguilla and the BVI, including that loans offered for reconstruction had strings attached (Pinkerton & Benwell, 2017). A BVI legislator likened the requirements to 'economic slavery' (Silva, 2018). In addition, the decision of the British Parliament to force the Caribbean OTs, but not the Crown Dependencies, to introduce stronger anti-money laundering laws caused further disquiet. Also, a controversial House of Commons Foreign Affairs Committee report that called for changes in areas such as same-sex marriage and reforming local OT citizenship was published in 2019 (Foreign Affairs Committee, 2019). Finally, and most recently, the decision of the Governor of the Cayman Islands to impose civil partnerships against the will of local politicians, and the suggestion that refugees entering Britain could be relocated 4000 miles to Ascension Island has raised alarm in the OTs about the lack of understanding and heavy-handedness by Britain. So, these broader strains in the OT–Britain relationship have shaped responses and reactions to the COVID-19 pandemic; most particularly in the BVI and the other Caribbean OTs. However, even where cooperation has been effective in Gibraltar, the Falklands, and to an extent Pitcairn, the events of the last few years will not be easily forgotten or forgiven.

Conclusion

Fortunately, at least for now, the four territories have controlled the spread of COVID-19, with the Falkland Islands having only a dozen cases in the resident population and Pitcairn no cases at all. Each territory has undertaken its role in a measured way to stem the spread, although the economic costs of the lockdown have been significant. Britain has afforded some assistance to all four territories, but there have been tensions, particularly with the BVI, and it does appear that Britain has taken a more benevolent attitude to the Falkland Islands and Gibraltar than to their more troublesome brethren in the Caribbean. There is a feeling, rightly or wrongly, in the BVI and other Caribbean OTs that skin colour does make a difference in how they are treated. As a result, there are increasing calls to look again at the constitutional relationship, including in the BVI and Bermuda; while the Cayman Islands has recently secured several amendments to its constitution (Connolly, 2020). Isolation is also an important theme. In some respects, it has had a beneficial effect, but key transportation links have been disrupted making it more difficult to organise medical treatment and the return of residents. In addition, geo-political concerns have been highlighted, but in contrasting ways. Gibraltar and Spain have worked well together, but relations between the Falkland Islands and Argentina remain frozen. Also, fear of 'the other' or those with suspected COVID-19 has been a theme in BVI and Pitcairn. Efforts have been made to limit the reach of these views, but they are clearly detrimental and will damage both monitoring and economic recovery efforts. In many respects, but perhaps not surprisingly, the pandemic has reinforced the strengths and weaknesses of the economic models being followed by the territories, the geo-strategic approaches they are taking, and their ties with Britain.

Disclosure statement

No potential conflict of interest was reported by the authors.

References

Ahmed, Z. (2020a, May 16). *Guv: Fiscal protocols aren't blocking Covid stimulus. The BVI Beacon.* https://www.bvibeacon.com/guv-fiscal-protocols-arent-blocking-covid-stimulus/

Ahmed, Z. (2020b, June 4). *$69.2m stimulus package unveiled. The BVI Beacon.* https://www.bvibeacon.com/62-9m-stimulus-package-unveiled/

Benwell, M. C., & Pinkerton, A. (2016). Brexit and the British Overseas Territories. *The RUSI Journal, 161*(4), 8–14. https://doi.org/10.1080/03071847.2016.1224489

Byron, J. (2019, April). Relations with the European Union and the United Kingdom Post-BREXIT: Perspectives from the Caribbean. *Études Caribéennes, 42*, 14705. https://doi.org/10.4000/etudescaribeennes.14705

Calder, S. (2020, August 27) *Quarantine: Gibraltar asks for leniency as UK government prepares to extend self-isolation rules. Independent.* https://www.independent.co.uk/travel/news-and-advice/gibraltar-coronavirus-quarantine-uk-germany-a9690816.html

Cavilla, C. (2020, March 23). *GHA now has 50 ventilators and is seeking more. Gibraltar Chronicle.* https://www.chronicle.gi/gha-now-has-50-ventilators-and-is-seeking-more/

Clegg, P. (2016). Brexit and the overseas territories: Repercussions for the periphery. *The Round Table: Commonwealth Journal of International Affairs, 105*(5), 543–556. https://doi.org/10.1080/00358533.2016.1229420

Clegg, P. (2018). The United Kingdom and its overseas territories: No longer a 'benevolent patron'? *Small States & Territories, 1*(2), 149–168. https://www.um.edu.mt/library/oar/handle/123456789/44833

CNW. (2020, September 26). *BVI Governor invites British Navy to secure borders; overrides premier. Caribbean National Weekly.* https://www.caribbeannationalweekly.com/caribbean-breaking-news-featured/bvi-governor-invities-british-navy-to-secure-borders-overrides-premier/

Connolly, N. (2020, November 12). *Privy Council approves constitutional changes. Cayman Compass.* https://www.caymancompass.com/2020/11/12/privy-council-approves-constitutional-changes/

Department of Transport. (2021, January 14). *Coronavirus (COVID-19): Travel corridors.* https://www.gov.uk/guidance/coronavirus-covid-19-travel-corridors

Dollimore, L. (2020, March 3). *Breaking: Coronavirus arrives in Gibraltar as patient tests positive after returning from Italy via Malaga Airport. The Olive Press.* https://www.theolivepress.es/spain-news/2020/03/03/breaking-coronavirus-arrives-in-gibraltar-as-patient-tests-positive-after-returning-from-italy-via-malaga-airport/

Falkland Islands Government. (2020, September 9). *COVID-19: Information and Guidance. 30 April.* https://fig.gov.fk/covid-19/public-updates/64-30-april-2020-covid-19-public-update

Filho, W., Lütz, J., Sattler, D., & Nunn, D. (2020). Coronavirus: COVID-19 Transmission in Pacific Small Island developing states. *International Journal of Environmental Research and Public Health, 17*(15), 5409. https://doi.org/10.3390/ijerph17155409

Foreign & Commonwealth Office (2020, June 10). *UK supports overseas territories in coronavirus (COVID-19) battle.* https://www.gov.uk/government/news/uk-supports-overseas-territories-in-coronavirus-covid-19-battle

Foreign Affairs Committee. (2019). *Global Britain and the British Overseas Territories: Resetting the relationship.* Fifteenth Report of Session 2017-19, House of Commons, HC 1464. https://publications.parliament.uk/pa/cm201719/cmselect/cmfaff/1464/1464.pdf

GBC. (2020, March 31). *Military help with Nightingale Field Hospital logistics.* https://www.gbc.gi/news/military-help-nightingale-field-hospital-logistics%C2%A0

Haynes, D. (2020, April 4). *Coronavirus: British serviceperson is Falkland Islands' first case of COVID-19. Sky News.* https://news.sky.com/story/coronavirus-british-serviceperson-is-falkland-islands-first-case-of-covid-19-11968338

HM Government of Gibraltar. (2020a, September 9). *Covid-19 public notifications' (Coronavirus statistics).* https://www.gibraltar.gov.gi/covid19

HM Government of Gibraltar. (2020b, May 12). *Unlock the Rock Part 1: A route map out of lockdown & starting to end confinement.* https://www.gibraltar.gov.gi/press-releases/unlock-the-rock-part-1-a-route-map-out-of-lockdown-starting-to-end-confinement-may-2020-5886

ITV News. (2020, April 1). *Gibraltar doctor hopes planning is putting off 'tidal wave' of coronavirus patients.* https://www.itv.com/news/2020-04-01/gibraltar-doctor-hopes-planning-is-putting-off-tidal-wave-of-coronavirus-patients

Kampa, D. (2020, May 28). *Premier, governor trade jabs over Protocols. The BVI Beacon.* https://www.bvibeacon.com/premier-governor-trade-jabs-over-protocols/

McGrath, C. (2020, March 26). *'Ticking time bomb' British territories bracing for coronavirus crisis – 250,000 at risk. Daily Express.* https://www.express.co.uk/news/world/1260874/coronavirus-news-falklands-gibraltar-covid-19-pandemic-british-territories

MercoPress. (2020a, May 8). *Governor praises the admirable public sector of the Falkland Islands.* https://en.mercopress.com/2020/05/08/governor-praises-the-admirable-public-sector-of-the-falkland-islands

MercoPress. (2020b, July 17). *Falklands' seafood industry faces environment of uncertainty.* https://en.mercopress.com/2020/07/17/falklands-seafood-industry-faces-environment-of-uncertainty

MercoPress. (2020c, August 28). *Falklands/Chile LATAM link remains suspended until at least January 2021.* https://en.mercopress.com/2020/08/28/falklands-chile-latam-link-remains-suspended-until-at-least-january-2021

Ministry of Defence. (2020, May 19). *UK Armed Forces step up support to the Caribbean Overseas Territories during coronavirus pandemic.* https://www.gov.uk/government/news/uk-armed-forces-step-up-support-to-the-caribbean-overseas-territories-during-coronavirus-pandemic

Montegriffo, M. (2020, June 14). How solidarity crossed the border in Corona-Hit Gibraltar, *Jacobin Magazine.* https://jacobinmag.com/2020/06/gibraltar-spain-coronavirus

Murphy, M., Jeyaseelan, S., Howitt, C., Greaves, N., Harewood, H., Quimby, K. R., Sobers, N., Landis, R. C., Rocke, K. D., & Hambleton, I. R. (2020, December). COVID-19 containment in

the Caribbean: The experience of small island developing states. *Research in Globalization, 2*, 100019. https://doi.org/10.1016/j.resglo.2020.100019
Nugent, C. (2020, March 27). *Isolation helped these islands delay a COVID-19 outbreak. Now, being remote could be their biggest problem. Time*. https://time.com/5811309/coronavirus-falklands/
Penguin News. (2020, November 13). *Two civilian COVID-19 cases identified in the Falklands*. 32(15). https://penguin-news.com/full-paper/2020/full-paper-20201113/
PIC. (2020b, March 12). *Minutes of the GPI workshop Le Soleal visit*. http://www.government.pn/minutes/Approved%20Le%20Soleal%20Council%20Workshop%20March%2012th%202020.pdf
PIC. (2020c, March 12). *Minutes of the GPI Corona virus management development protocol workshop*. http://www.government.pn/minutes/Approved%20Corona%20Virus%20Management%20Protocols%20Council%20Workshop%2012th%20March%202020.pdf
PIC. (2020d, March 30/31). *Minutes of the GPI Corona virus management development protocol workshop II and III notes*. http://www.government.pn/minutes/Approved%20Corona%20Virus%20Management%20Protocols%20Workshops%2030th%20&%2031st%20of%20March%202020.pdf
PIC. (2020e, April 8). *Public meeting notes: COVID-19 management protocols*. http://www.government.pn/minutes/Approved%20Public%20Meeting%20Notes%208th%20April%202020
PIC. (2020f, April 14). *Minutes of the regular council meeting held at the public hall*. http://www.government.pn/minutes/Approved%20Regular%20Council%20Meeting%20Minutes%2014th%20April%202020.pdf
PIC. (2020g, May 21). *Minutes of the special council meeting held at the public hall*. http://www.government.pn/minutes/Approved%20Special%20Council%20Meeting%20Minutes%2021st%20May%202020.pdf
PIC. (2020h, July 15). *Minutes of the regular council meeting held at the public hall*. http://www.government.pn/minutes/Approved%20Regular%20Council%20Minutes%2015th%20July%202020.pdf
PIC. (2020i, July 30). *Public meeting notes: COVID-19 management protocols*. http://www.government.pn/minutes/Approved%20Public%20Meeting%20Notes%2030th%20July%202020.pdf
PIC (Pitcairn Island Council). (2020a, March 10). *Minutes of the public meeting held at the public hall*. http://www.government.pn/minutes/APPROVED%20Council%20minutes%2029th%20March%202017.pdf
Picardo, F. (2020, March 18). https://twitter.com/FabianPicardo/status/1240262694269259776
Pinkerton, A., & Benwell, M. C. (2017, September 11). *Hurricane Irma's devastation of Caribbean territories piles pressure on strained relationship with UK. The Conversation*. https://theconversation.com/hurricane-irmas-devastation-of-caribbean-territories-piles-pressure-on-strained-relationship-with-uk-83833
Silva, K. (2018, April 11). *BVI still reeling from 2017 hurricane season. Cayman Compass*. https://www.caymancompass.com/2018/04/11/bvi-still-reeling-from-2017-hurricane-season/
Smith, J. (2020, April 15). *Gibraltar can now produce its own Oxygen for Hospital and no longer needs to Import from Spain. EuroWeekly News*. https://www.euroweeklynews.com/2020/04/15/gibraltar-can-now-produce-its-own-oxygen-for-hospital-use-and-no-longer-needs-to-import-from-spain/
Télam. (2020, April 12). *Contabilizar a los habitantes de Malvinas es un hecho de soberanía*. dijo intendente de Río Grande. https://www.telam.com.ar/notas/202004/451002-contabilizar-a-los-habitantes-de-malvinas-es-un-hecho-de-soberania-dijo-intendente-de-rio-grande.html
The House of Assembly of the Virgin Islands. (2020) *Resolution No. 16 of 2020, Gazetted 13 August*. https://www.bvibeacon.com/wp-content/uploads/2020/09/Resolution-No.-16-of-2020-SAP-No.-1-of-2020.pdf
Thomas, D. (2020, May 13). *Gibraltar hopes to the be the first country in the world to do Covid-19 antibody tests on entire population. The Olive Press*. https://www.theolivepress.es/spain-news/2020/05/13/gibraltar-hopes-to-be-first-country-to-do-covid-19-antibody-tests-on-entire-population/

Waldinger, J. (2020a, September 4). *Beefed up border patrol nabs boat. The BVI Beacon.* https://www.bvibeacon.com/border-patrol-nabs-boat/

Waldinger, J. (2020b, October 2). *Governor Gus Jaspert enlists Royal Navy for border security. The BVI Beacon.* https://www.bvibeacon.com/governor-border-security/

Wheatley, B. (2020, June 3). *Commentary - Covid-19 compared to hurricanes. The BVI Beacon.* https://www.bvibeacon.com/commentary-covid-19-compared-to-hurricanes/

Wintour, P. (2021, January 18). British Virgin Island governor launches inquiry into alleged corruption. *The Guardian.* https://www.theguardian.com/world/2021/jan/18/uk-launches-inquiry-alleged-corruption-british-virgin-island

Yusuf, H. O., & Chowdhury, T. (2019). The persistence of colonial constitutionalism in British Overseas Territories. *Global Constitutionalism*, *8*(1), 157–190. https://doi.org/10.1017/S2045381718000369

Index

Note: Page numbers in **bold** refer to tables and those in *italics* refer to figures.

For Product Safety Concerns and Information please contact our EU
representative GPSR@taylorandfrancis.com
Taylor & Francis Verlag GmbH, Kaufingerstraße 24, 80331 München, Germany

www.ingramcontent.com/pod-product-compliance
Ingram Content Group UK Ltd.
Pitfield, Milton Keynes, MK11 3LW, UK
UKHW052211190926
475702UK00006B/970

* 9 7 8 1 0 3 2 3 7 6 6 6 0 *